I'VE NEVER LOVED HIM MORE

Candy Abbott writes not only from her experience and her heart but from her connection with God. What ends up on the page is amazing in its honesty, astonishing in its wisdom, and authentic in its wit—even in the midst of tears. If you love someone suffering from dementia, sit down with this book. You will stand up at the end, ready to apply Candy's soul knowledge to your own journey. I know I am.

—Nancy Rue
Best-selling fiction author

I've Never Loved Him More is a very heartfelt, personal, and readable book about caring for and loving someone with Alzheimer's dementia. It will make you laugh and cry. Everyone who has or had a loved one who suffers from some form of dementia needs to read this book. When I came to the part about 1 Corinthians 13, I thought, *Candy is a living example of the Love Chapter.* This book contains a message that most of our world needs to hear.

—Dave Kelly, BSW
Harrison Senior Living, Dementia Units

Look no further for a transparent companion with whom you can navigate the mysteries of Alzheimer's and dementia. Candy Abbott's words and word pictures offer a written preservation of love's offerings even in the face of monumental change. This is not a capricious diary but rather a contemplative chronicle of a wife's incremental acceptance of her husband as he was and the man he has become. For couples about to marry as well as those married for years, this is compulsory reading. *I've Never Loved Him More* paints a beautiful and brutally honest reality of what it takes to keep the vow "until death do us part."

—Chris Ann Waters
Author, Speaker, Bereavement Specialist, and Hospice Chaplain
Seasons of Goodbye: Working Your Way Through Loss

Thank you and God bless you, Candy, for opening the door to your home and your heart. Your words are poignant, powerful, and practical. This is a must-read for anyone caring for a spouse who has Alzheimer's as well as for family and friends.

—Marlene Bagnull
Author and Conference Director

Candy's book pierces my heart on two levels: first, the up-close-and-personal intimate details of caring for a radically changed husband with God's patience and humor; and secondly, a personal, holy nudge for me to respond with equal kindness and grace to the simple frustrations of daily living with my own husband. With great wisdom, Candy breathes life into a humanly impossible situation by reminding us that with God, all things are possible. Instead of grudgingly resigning herself to serve Drew ("I *have* to do this for him"), she demonstrates God's perspective of unending love, no matter what the cost ("I *get* to do this for him").

—Sara Lewis
Fruitbearer author of the Called to Pray series

In *I've Never Loved Him More*, Candy Abbott chronicles her husband's journey from a healthy adult male into the beginning of his mid-stage Alzheimer's disease. She captures (in great detail) the profound impact this disease has on family members as well as vividly describing her new role as a caregiver. Her insightful writings are full of excellent ideas and suggestions for others who have been thrust into this role. She is uniquely able to combine humor, reality, and strong faith to maintain a loving relationship with her husband as he slowly declines over the years. Delaware Hospice is both honored and pleased to help both husband and wife as they progress on this journey. We will continue to support Candy through our Transitions Program and through other programs and services as needs arise. We highly recommend this book to all who are dealing with this terrible disease or a serious illness of any kind.

—Al Morris, MS
Senior Transitions Coordinator
Delaware Hospice

I found your story both heart-wrenching and heart-warming. You are a remarkable example of how to honor one's marriage vows. I truly enjoyed reading the book and feel as though I have a whole new insight on what it's like to be a caregiver. It's really well done.

—Michele Procino-Wells, Esquire
Procino-Wells & Woodland, LLC

Perhaps one of the most difficult and heartbreaking issues I faced in more than twenty-five years in the United Methodist pastorate is the descent brought on by Alzheimer's. It is evil and insidious, totally robbing its victims of their identity. What a helpless feeling the affected, their families, and loved ones experience as they watch this scourge decimate mental awareness, memory, and social skills. "Who is this person?" is a question asked over and over. What's worse is when the loved one looks at his or her wife, husband, or children and asks repeatedly, "Who are you?" There are no cures, as yet, and only minimal medications can delay or lessen symptoms.

But, take heart, folks. There is a new and encouraging resource in (my friend) Candy Abbott's new book, *I've Never Loved Him More*. Demonstrating an unwavering reliance on her faith and deep relationship with God, this book is an intimate portrait of the journey she and her beloved husband, Drew, are taking through their encounter with his disease. It is a missal of love written deeply from the heart and by the Spirit of God. Candy openly shares how her Lord directs them through the darkness and despair of Alzheimer's into pockets of Light. See what they have faced, along with what has worked and what has not.

This book is such a gift and so refreshing. I truly believe it has the power to become a new standard reference for the Alzheimer's community. God bless it and those to whom some light dawns, my friend.

—Rev. Carol E. Svecz
Pastor/Elder, United Methodist Church

I've Never Loved Him More

A Husband's Alzheimer's.

A Wife's Devotion.

CANDY ABBOTT

FRUITBEARER PUBLISHING LLC

Copyright © 2017 Candy Abbott
ISBN 978-1-938796-08-1
Library of Congress Control Number: 2017900356
SAN 920-380X
ISNI 0000 0000 5048 9968

Health/Diseases: Alzheimer's Disease • Christian/Family & Relationships
• Christian/Inspirational

Nancy Rue, Content Editor
Fran D. Lowe, Copy Editor

Cover photo by Dana Abbott Painter (Drew's daughter)
taken in Bermuda on John Smith's Bay

Published by Fruitbearer Publishing, LLC
P.O. Box 777 • Georgetown, DE 19947
302.856.6649 • FAX 302.856.7742
www.fruitbearer.com • info@fruitbearer.com

Printed in the United States of America

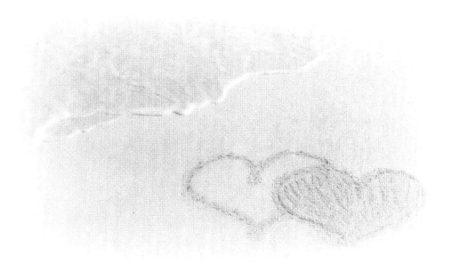

To Drew, of course,

WHO WILL NEVER READ THIS BOOK
BUT WOULDN'T EXPECT ANYTHING LESS THAN
HOW TRANSPARENT I'VE BEEN WITH OUR LIVES
BECAUSE HE KNOWS ME SO WELL.

There is no substitute
for the love
of an Alzheimer's caregiver.

— Bob DeMarco
AlzheimersReadingRoom.com

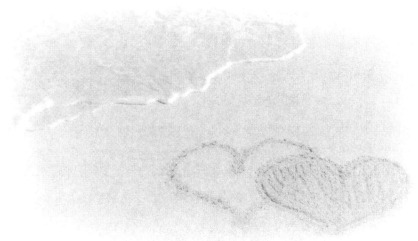

Contents

Foreword

I met Candy Abbott at an Alzheimer's support group in a quiet room at Harrison House in Georgetown, Delaware, a senior living community. She and I had an immediate spiritual connection that was so compelling it gave me goosebumps. I couldn't stop looking at her because the light in her eyes shone with the very grace of God. I sat and listened to Candy's story about her journey as a wife and caregiver to her loving, kind, gentle husband who has Alzheimer's disease. I have attended many support groups in my career as a community relations coordinator in home health care. Never have I encountered a more loving, kind family that is so supportive of one other. I knew from that moment that Candy and I were going to become fast friends.

I've Never Loved Him More is a chronological journey into the unknown and sometimes scary, dark world of Alzheimer's disease. Yet, this book is anything but dark and scary. Instead, it is delightful, funny, and heartwarming.

Best-selling author Nancy Rue says, "Like the true storyteller she is, Candy spins the funny scenes in a way that brings on the belly laughter, sometimes in the midst of tears. It's never forced. It's never inappropriate. It's just true wit born out of a cheerful spirit that cannot be daunted by even this long, trying ordeal."

My personal favorite is the Bermuda chapter where Candy tells the "underwear story" that happened during their fortieth anniversary cruise. Once you read the episode by the coral reef and the turquoise waters, you'll be echoing Candy's words, "Have I got a story for you!"

Nancy also says, "With her use of Scripture throughout the pages, Candy doesn't ask the reader to simply read the passages and have faith. Instead, she explains in a practical, concrete way just how those verses work in a life that's being put through the refining fire. Writing truth from a place of authenticity, she speaks in simple terms to the person who is emotionally writhing, offering the benefit of her hard-won wisdom and experience without ever being condescending. She owns her mistakes as well as triumphs."

The dialogue throughout the book demonstrates the relationship Candy and Drew have built over the years and how a home filled with patience, loving kindness, and understanding has equipped Candy to be the caregiver her husband needs, wants, and trusts.

Candy's journey with Alzheimer's offers a vision of hope—the light in the tunnel, not at the end of the tunnel. This book truly delivers!

Cindy Broschart
Alzheimer's Advocate and
Home Health Care Community Relations Coordinator

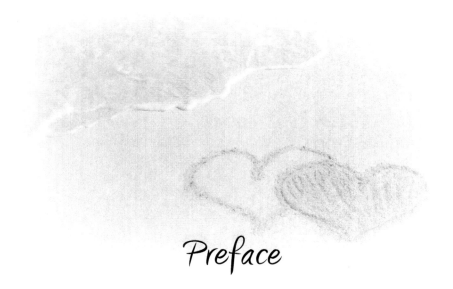

Preface

When I first stepped into the mind-boggling world of Alzheimer's with my beloved husband, my daughter and several friends said, "You should write a book." Each time, I recoiled at the thought because it was all I could do to get through every day juggling my ever increasing responsibilities. "I have to live it before I can write it," I told them.

And then Nancy Rue, my writing mentor, suggested that it might be therapeutic for me to "capture some scenes." Right from the beginning, my manuscript began teaching me things about myself as I recorded my raw emotions and the mysterious changes taking place in Drew.

Before long, my motivation shifted to helping others as I typed daily snippets of my fears, successes, missteps, and downright funny incidents. In the second year of my life as an "open book," I began thinking ahead and contemplating which responses to Drew's changing behavior would show moral courage and serve as good examples for my readers (instead of knee jerk reactions).

So, thank you, dear reader, for impacting the quality of life in the Abbott household. In turn, I hope these pages help you, too.

To realize the worth of an anchor,
we need to feel the stress of the storm.

—Anonymous

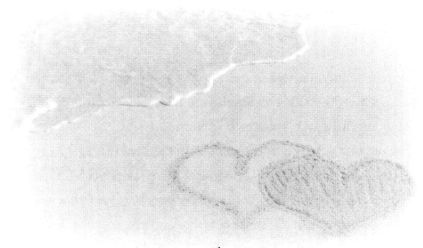

Introduction

Love . . . always protects, always trusts, always hopes, always perseveres. Love never fails.

—1 Corinthians 13:7-8 (NIV)

These words are spoken at many a wedding. But living them out is easier said than done. When Candy and Drew Abbott took their vows in 1975, they did not expect dementia to take away the memory of those vows for Drew. *I've Never Loved Him More* chronicles how 1 Corinthians looks on a daily basis through the lens of Alzheimer's. It has taken patience, endurance, creativity, humor, Christian faith, prayers, and a whole lot of fortitude supplied by God to meet the demands and adjustments of this memory-stealing and life-altering disease.

When you enter this book, you enter the Abbott home and become a part of the household dynamics. Candy describes the days, leaving out no details. Written in journal format, each day is different and illustrative of the *bears all things* characteristic of love. Drew's repetitive questions, the oddities of not being able to carry out simple tasks such as feeding the dog and picking up Cokes at the store—all the nuances of memory loss—are clearly documented. These seemingly routine examples of daily life take on a different flavor when Alzheimer's claims cognition.

For anyone who has or is coping with the strain of caregiving for a loved one with dementia or Alzheimer's, this book provides a friend in Candy on this unpredictable journey. As she cares for Drew, she uses her journal entries to mark the emotional and physical challenges that ensue, and connects the reader with possibilities to make this journey not only bearable but redeemable.

Since God can use anything, Candy believes that God will use this experience in their marriage as a chart for others as they, too, navigate the maze of memory loss. Furthermore, Candy's journal entries of changes in Drew allowed her to record the memories they are still making together. In this way, writing has been for Candy a therapeutic and cathartic mechanism toward the acceptance of this irreversible disease. Writing can be so for anyone who will take the time to write out their journey.

Buckle up for honesty. Candy is as transparent as glass about their marriage. This transparency includes everything from finances to sexuality. Her warmth, humor, logic, and gift for writing make this a readable record as well as an open invitation to the heart of this marriage. With all the difficulties they have faced, Candy has succeeded in threading respect and dignity for Drew into each page. Alzheimer's took memory, but it cannot take love. Candy strives to honor her husband—no matter what. For Drew, his episodes of cerebral weakness do not stop the intermittent return of recognizing Candy as the one who brings him peace. That remembrance is more than enough to continue to carry him through another day of unknowns, and gives Candy a measure of encouragement to keep them both moving forward.

There is no logical conclusion for those who suffer with Alzheimer's. Research continues, and hope is employed for those who bear the disease and those who care for them. Candy provides resources at the end of this book, and readers will gain new information to apply to respective needs. The bulk of information, however, rests in these personal pages of truth about the ins and outs of living life with grace and kindness in the face of a disease that robs. Grace replenishes. That is what Candy believes God has done for her and Drew and can do for others. This book is proof of replenishment.

First Lady Eleanor Roosevelt said of herself, "I am my husband's legs." In this book, Candy is her husband's mind. She remembers for him and for readers the years of their lives, spotlighting memories and untangling mental yarns for Drew and for us. This volume does not gloss over the frustration and myriad emotions associated with the incremental and fluid onset of the disease. However, it does portray recognition of and respect for all that has been and seeks to convey gratitude for the years that were lived in the fullness of memory and health.

"Have I Told You Lately That I Love You" by Rod Stewart is on Candy and Drew's playlist. So is "Only You" by The Platters. By the end of this book, you will be able to see that love is not always estimated in words, but in actions too. Candy tells Drew she loves him by fulfilling caring acts when he does not even know what she is doing for him and when he sometimes forgets who she is. In return, when Drew does recognize Candy and he wants and needs her near him, he continues to say with his heart, *only you*.

Dementia and Alzheimer's make for a strange path of mystery. While this book is written by a wife about a husband, its readership is anyone who wants to understand more about what it means to love someone—anyone—when memory is weakened or lost. It is especially beneficial reading for those considering marriage, for it does not sanitize the physical unknowns and emotional complexities down the road. Romance has its place, but marriage has its purpose. It is not for weaklings, as *I've Never Loved Him More* describes.

Sit back, digest, and lean into this book with an open heart. As you do, you are certain to reach the final page with a renewed value for time, life, and the relationships you hold dear—or the relationships you want to hold dear while there is time to do so.

This book provides a frontal view of the fragility of time. It allows an encounter with the truth that tomorrow is not promised. Therefore, live today in all its routine, beauty, responsibilities, and scope of possibility while there is time. God bless and be with you in this reading, and always.

Chris Ann Waters
Author, *Seasons of Goodbye:*
Working Your Way Through Loss
Hospice Chaplain

CHAPTER ONE

The Way We Were

The instant Drew wrapped his arms around me, my racing heart settled into a steady beat. Moments before, we had been sprinting around together from room to room with my checklist and then carrying boxes, suitcases, posters, and registration packets to the car. Now that everything had been loaded into the trunk and back seat of the Camry, it was time to say goodbye as we always did before one of my events—standing together in the living room with him holding me close.

The aroma of lilacs from outside lingered around us as I closed my eyes and nestled my head into his neck and shoulder. The room was silent except for the ticking of the clock on the mantel. He spoke, and the sound of his voice vibrated with authority in my ears and in my chest.

"Master," he prayed, "Candy is heading out once again to do Your work. She has put a lot into this weekend, and a lot of nice ladies are coming. Let it be good for everybody. Give Candy peace." He paused. "And confidence. Most of all, keep her safe and bring her back to me. Amen."

Simple words. Powerful words. Loving words.

In our entire marriage, I have always felt that Drew loved me more than I loved him. I know you can't measure love, but the word "supportive" in the dictionary should have "Drew Abbott" as the definition. Until the last decade or so, we both held full-time jobs, but I was often preoccupied with the kids' homework, after-school activities, and meal planning; immersed in writing books and publishing for others; attending choir rehearsals, leading Bible studies, or teaching Sunday school. It seemed like I was always dashing out the door for an appointment or a meeting and giving him a quick hug and kiss.

He, on the other hand, was always thinking ahead to make sure I had everything I needed (gas, money, a helping hand, a night out) and gave me his full attention when I got home. He was quick with compliments. He saw needs and filled them without fanfare. He did the laundry, cleaned up the kitchen, and kept us supplied with bread and milk. He was as good a father to my daughter as he was to his own children. He took care of the vehicles, finances, and lawn. Filled with an extra measure of common sense and intuition about which situations or people might be toxic to me, he served as my constant sounding board. As the kids grew up and began having children of their own, he continued as our family anchor and encourager.

Thirty-five years into our marriage, all that began to change. You'll see as you read on that a terrible disease crept into our home and changed that dynamic completely. It could have torn us apart, and yet it is turning out so differently. I want to share the story that led me to be able to say, "I've never loved him more."

In a society that is becoming increasingly filled with noncommittal, "what's-in-it-for-me?" relationships, some spouses run from stressors like Alzheimer's, spouting, "I didn't sign on for this," or "I want to remember him as he was."

Even those who choose to stay may view the whole ordeal through a negative lens, so they are left with a sad, bitter experience. People with Alzheimer's, sensitized to emotions, often serve as mirrors by reflecting the mood of their caregivers who would be better served by guarding their peace and intentionally setting a softer tone.

And then there are those like me, steadfast for the duration, who discover the depth of what the apostle Paul meant when he said in Acts 20:35 (NIV), "In everything I did, I showed you that by this kind of hard work we must help the weak, remembering the words the Lord Jesus himself said: 'It is more blessed to give than to receive.'"

My Alzheimer's journey with Drew is indeed "hard work," but the experience is changing me for the better. Of all the previous ministries I have poured myself into, none have given me the depth of satisfaction I find in ministering to the man I became one with in 1975. He is growing increasingly weak, but I am growing increasingly strong because of the truth of Philippians 4:13 (NKJV): "I can do all things through Christ who strengthens me."

If you or someone you know has been pulled into the surreal world of caring for a loved one who has become a ghost of his or her former self, I hope that my bumps and dents can translate into a reminder to dig deeper to find an extra measure of kindness, gentleness, or humor in your day.

Let these pages serve as an eye-opener to live in the moment. After all, this moment—this very moment—is all we really have. See that? This moment has now become that moment, gone forever.

"Feelings are everywhere—be gentle."

— J. Masai

CHAPTER TWO

An Unwelcome Surprise

November 2010

It all began with the discovery of what was described as "an incidental finding." On Drew's first visit to the vascular surgeon, Dr. Katz ran a routine carotid artery CT brain scan to check for any sign of possible stroke activity. That part looked fine, but he was surprised and alarmed to find a sizeable tumor in the left frontal lobe. He contacted our primary care physician right away, and Dr. Palekar's office called us in for an urgent appointment. After breaking the news as gently as possible, he recommended a neurosurgeon affiliated with Christiana Care Hospital.

"Dr. Sugarman is very good and in high demand," Dr. Palekar told us, "so it's hard to get an appointment, but I'll see what I can do."

Dr. Sugarman's office called the next day with an opening in three weeks. We were shopping at Sam's Club when my cell phone rang. Drew held our ice cream cup while I talked with the nurse and rummaged through my purse to find my calendar. When I hung up, I remember feeling equally relieved and anxious to schedule the appointment, maybe because I had been holding my breath most of the time.

December 2010

When the day of the appointment arrived, I drove because Drew seemed nervous enough without having to navigate through traffic on Route 1 to find the Delaware Neurological Group in Newark. We had to wait about an hour (that's why they call it a "waiting room"), and I kept reminding him how fortunate we were to even get an appointment.

The staff was professional and courteous. Dr. Sugarman had a wonderful bedside manner, which was especially good for Drew.

After reviewing the scans, he explained what a meningioma was and said we were fortunate to find the tumor before there were any symptoms.

"It's not malignant and is located just beneath the skull and not inside your brain, so this will be a simple operation. I think we can get you scheduled before Christmas."

"Whoa, not so fast," Drew said. He didn't relish having his head opened up, and for good reason. "My dad had Parkinson's and *died* from brain surgery. Unless it's absolutely necessary, I don't want it."

After Dr. Sugarman had asked about the details, he said, "Two things: First, the kind of surgery your dad had was deep in the brain and very different from yours, which is easily accessible. Second, it was done in 1968, and the medical profession has come a long way since then."

But Drew would not be persuaded, so Dr. Sugarman proposed we "keep an eye on it" with MRIs every three to six months.

At the time, avoiding surgery seemed good to me, too. Now, years later, I'm wondering if we could have avoided Alzheimer's altogether. But this I *do* know: we honored Drew's wishes and made the best decision we knew to make at the time.

March and September 2011

The MRIs from both visits were consistent with the initial one. No change, praise God! We left the office feeling optimistic and celebrated over lunch at a nearby steakhouse.

April 2012

A couple of years later, I began noticing subtle changes in Drew's memory. He kept forgetting to buckle his seatbelt, a regular habit he used to be adamant about. And there were other little things, like losing interest in the men's group that met at McDonald's every morning and being more argumentative than usual. It wasn't enough to send up any red flags, but I began to suspect something was off-kilter that may have been caused by the tumor.

At our next appointment with Dr. Sugarman, the MRI showed that the tumor hadn't grown, and I didn't think to mention anything about his memory.

During the following visit six months later, I told Dr. Sugarman about my concerns but couldn't recall anything specific.

"There's nothing wrong with my memory," Drew insisted. "You're the one who keeps misplacing things."

Dr. Sugarman said that the tumor shouldn't affect his memory because of where it was located, but the edema from it could be putting pressure on that area of the brain. In front of Drew, he suggested I keep a log of specific situations so we could see if there was a pattern. I was relieved to have something tangible to do that would provide proof.

Drew was understandably defensive. "So you're going to be watching my every move, trying to catch me doing something you can write down?"

The doctor saved me from having to answer by leaning forward and looking at Drew with compassion. "She's going to do what I'm suggesting because she cares about you. MRIs can't tell me everything I need to know about what's going on with your tumor. Symptoms are subtle, and the best way to detect if there is pressure on your brain is to record any unusual incidents so I can make an informed evaluation."

July 16, 2013

For our next appointment, I brought three copies of the following log with me so Drew and I could follow along as Dr. Sugarman looked it over:

January – July 2013

- Slower movement when eating. Fork to mouth sometimes seems like slow motion, which might be a good thing because he eats less. Has been losing weight and Dr. Palekar is pleased with that. His lab results are excellent on all counts, and his blood pressure is perfect.

- Driving habits are changing. When turning off the highway, instead of moving to the right so traffic can pass, he slows way down and complains about people hugging his bumper. Sometimes they beep their horn, which irritates him.

- He poked along at 15 mph looking for the turn for our daughter's street and would have missed it if I hadn't pointed it out.

- When going to restaurants we frequent in nearby towns, he knows the general vicinity but can't remember where to turn. Lately, I've been offering to drive, and he's fine with that.

- Didn't remember that he has used Quicken for taxes for the past five years. I reinstalled the program on his new computer so he could do our taxes, but it looked foreign to him, so he did everything by hand this year.

- When my 1099 came in from my pension, I gave it to Drew and mentioned that it was important for taxes and to put it in a "safe place," but he didn't know where it was when the accountant asked for it. I eventually found it on the sewing machine.

- He sleeps well, but his habits are changing. He used to fall asleep around 9:00 after watching TV but is staying up later (11:00 or sometimes midnight) and waking in the morning around 9:00 instead of 5:30, which used to be typical.

- A delightful new occurrence: he sings happy little songs from childhood, i.e., "I've Been Working on the Railroad" and "She'll Be Comin' 'Round the Mountain."

- He sometimes tells waitresses that he is ready to pay the bill and insists that they wait while he s-l-o-w-l-y counts out the money.

- Our eye doctor expressed concern that Drew couldn't remember we've been tracking beginning signs of macular degeneration and cataracts for some years. Drew told Dr.

Robinson, "You must have me confused with my brother, Howard, who has macular degeneration." Howard does have this problem, but the doctor wasn't at all confused.

- Confusion over how to serve communion in church. We had been given instructions on which aisle to serve, and instead of serving his assigned aisle, he followed me, creating some awkwardness for us as well as the congregation.

- His perception when parking the car is off (sometimes too far back, sometimes over the line, sometimes crooked), and he fusses with me if I point this out.

- Trash pick-up for recycling is every other week. In the car, I mentioned that we would need to put both receptacles out when we got home. At bedtime, I asked if he remembered and he said "yes." But the next day, I realized he had only taken one bin out to the curb. He insists I never mentioned both. This could be hearing-related or memory-related or both. The solution is to circle the calendar on the appropriate dates.

- He says I have been making negative remarks, which I guess I have, but I'm only trying to be helpful. If only he knew how many times I've held my tongue and ignored the changes I see in him. I will work on being more positive by acknowledging the many things he still does well and without fanfare: doing yard work, emptying the dishwasher, cleaning the bathroom, making the bed, shopping for groceries, picking up prescriptions, taking care of the cars, repairing brickwork on the front porch, feeding our dog and cat, etc.

- Bill paying has become confusing for him, so I help him on occasion by being more intentional about a place for mail that requires action.

All the way through the list, Drew argued that these things were not true—instead, I had exaggerated or made them up.

When we finished, I asked the doctor, "Is it possible we might be dealing with two things? The tumor and maybe some kind of dementia?"

"Well," Dr. Sugarman said, "it's possible. I could refer you to a neurologist for testing, but he would tell you that we first need to remove the tumor to make sure it's not the culprit."

I'm not even sure what was said or how Dr. Sugarman convinced Drew, but we left the office with surgery scheduled for August 28, 2013. This came more as a relief to me than a blow. He would have the surgery, and then he would be fine.

August 28, 2013

The surgery was successful. Following recovery, they placed him in a room in ICU that had a window by the nurses' station. That evening, while his daughter Dana, son Troy, and I were gathered around the bed, Drew even cracked a few jokes between mini-naps.

"You say funny things," Dana said. And then he would fall asleep again.

We talked softly until he stirred again. This time, he stared at a picture on the wall across from his bed and said, "Why is there a pig in the room?" There was no pig in the room, just a picture of the faces of a man and woman.

We laughed about the pig in the room and Drew picking at the air because he was trying to catch invisible bugs. Troy said he thought he was hallucinating, but we brushed it off as the aftermath of surgery.

Another patient's family members were milling around in the hallway, waiting their turn to visit in the room that was, no doubt, as small as ours. A bony man who was so wrinkled he must have been the great-great-grandfather slouched against the wall. I felt sorry for him. His dark face had sorrow etched in the crevasses, making him look, well . . . dreadful and older than old.

The next time Drew woke up, he glanced at the man in the hallway just in time to see him jump, double over, and scurry past the window as if he had a sharp pain and had to find a bathroom quick.

Drew whispered to me with fear in his eyes, "I just saw a demon."

I knew what he'd seen. The guy had all the characteristics of what you'd think a demon might look like—hunched frame, sunken cheeks, distorted facial expression, and bulging eyes. I cocked my head and said, "You just saw a what?"

"A demon."

Dana echoed my question. "Dad, what did you say?"

Drew's eyebrows knit together, and we waited for him to repeat it. Instead, he shook his head and said, "Never mind."

After our stressful day, Dana, Troy, and I laughed so hard that we cried. Drew was puzzled over what was so funny, and the more we tried to explain that he said he saw a demon but then thought he'd better not say so, the harder we laughed. Although he had no clue about what was so funny, he laughed right along with us.

August 31, 2013

I was just leaving the motel to go to the hospital when the nurse called to ask how soon I could get there. Apparently, they'd had "an incident," and Drew was asking when Candy would be there. He's always been a kind and gentle man, but the nurse told me he had almost pulled out his catheter and been so combative that morning it took four security guards to get him back to bed.

When I walked into the room, he was relaxed, and I congratulated myself for having such a calming influence. I convinced the nurse to untie the restraints they had on his wrists.

"They're mean to me," he said softly. "They won't let me go to the bathroom, and I have to pee."

"They're not mean, honey. You have a catheter that's catching the urine, so you need to stay in bed."

Moments later, he was struggling against me to get out of bed. His grip was strong, his eyes were wild, and his voice rose with every word. He got halfway to the bathroom dragging me along with him before the nurses and security guards were able to take over.

So they tied him to the rails again.

Drew glared at me with a look of betrayal. "You're my wife. You're supposed to help me. Why won't you help me?"

It was a long afternoon for me sitting there feeling like a bad wife.

Drew kept picking at the strips of cloth that bound him and finally pulled one loose just about the time our grandson, Trevor, arrived. I whispered what was going on, and he jumped right in.

"Here, Granddad," he said, "let me help you with that." And he retied it.

The next day when the doctors did their rounds, we discussed the drugs he was on—ones to keep the swelling down in the brain, along with anti-seizure medicine. One of them was Haldol, which makes some people delusional and combative. The doctor discontinued it at once, and Drew's confrontational behavior drained away, leaving me hopeful again. When we got him home and on the road to recovery, life could get back to normal.

October 2013

In the months it took him to recover, it seemed to all of us that his memory was improving, but maybe we saw what we wanted to see. Maybe we explained away too easily the memory glitches of a forgotten story that he used to enjoy telling over and over or a forgotten name of someone he should have known.

CHAPTER THREE

Shotgun Blast to Denial

January 6, 2014

When we met with Dr. Sugarman this time, he said Drew was healing well, and the MRI showed no sign of the tumor trying to come back. The next appointment was in six months, which suited me just fine. I could breathe again.

Or could I? Inside my "knower," I knew that something wasn't right.

April 2014

By April, the reality of what was happening hit me full force. The shotgun blast that blew away any lingering denial of Drew's condition came in the form of the stark reality of our finances.

From the beginning of our marriage, Drew has always done a masterful job of managing our household finances. Our rule of thumb was to put most of our expenses (gas, food, medicine) on credit cards so we'd have a record, and then pay them off completely each month. When the bills came, I routinely handed them over to him and never gave them another thought.

The first major blow was the time I tried to use our Master Card at the grocery store. It was declined.

"Try it again, please. It should be fine since we have a pretty high credit limit," I said.

The cashier tried it three times, but each time it was declined. *That's odd, because we had a $14,000 credit line. Must be a mistake.*

No mistake. It was maxed out. I used our Discover card.

That same day, the envelope from Discover came in the mail, and I thought I'd better open it instead of handing it to Drew like usual. My hands began to shake when I saw that the minimum payment for that month was $2,000-plus and then noticed we were dangerously close to our $18,000 limit on that card. It felt like someone reached into my chest and twisted my gut into a pretzel when I realized Drew hadn't been paying on any of the cards, which put us in the 29% interest category, so the balances were climbing exponentially. Feeling lightheaded, I had to grip the kitchen bar to steady myself.

About the time I was coming to grips with the whole scenario of losing him to "some sort of dementia," I suddenly had to take responsibility for not only handling but also straightening out our finances, which were now in shambles. In this case, ignorance was not bliss. It was devastating on so many levels, especially since I have an aversion to working with numbers in the first place.

The reality of my grief had been building up for days, even though I had held the tears and fears back as long as I could, to put on my happy face for Drew. But that day it needed to come out. He caught me staring out the window with tears welling in my eyes.

"What's the matter?" he asked.

The grief of not being able to tell my confidant and soul mate about this life-altering heartbreak threatened to consume me, but I plastered on a smile.

"Oh . . ." I searched my heart for a quick and satisfying reply. "I was just thinking about how much I love you, and it's pretty overwhelming sometimes."

April 10, 2014

I kept the tears bottled up inside for the next day or two—and then came Thursday. For more than eight years now, several women and I have met in the prayer room of my church every Thursday morning to spend an hour in praise and thanksgiving, confession and repentance, personal petition, intercession for others, and meditation and assessment. That day, it was all about *me*. I went early and sat alone with God and my thoughts. From the moment Wilmetta stepped into the room, I began sobbing and choked out the words I'd been rehearsing in my mind but dared not say aloud until now: "Drew has some sort of dementia."

Then Sharon arrived, and more tears and fears spilled out of me. "I'm losing him," I gasped between words, "and I don't know . . . what to do."

After receiving their counsel and comforting words, I bowed my head on an unseen altar in that little 12 x 12 room, a sacred space in my time of need. They laid their hands on my head and shoulders and prayed for me.

Sharon had to leave early to go to work, but Wilmetta stayed until I was able to collect myself. As we left, the pastor came out of his office, and all it took was one glance for him to ask, "What's wrong?" His advice was immediate and on the mark. "You are Drew's advocate," he said. "It's up to you to speak on his behalf and make decisions for him."

I couldn't go home to Drew with my eyes all puffy and red, so I drove around aimlessly praying, "Help me. Help me." And then more words came. "I'm scared, Lord. I feel so inadequate."

The Holy Spirit's gentle whisper spoke to my spirit. "Fear not, for I am with you. Moment by moment and day by day, I will show you what to do. First and foremost, your job is to love Drew." Immediately, a verse from the famous love chapter popped up in my mind: "Love is patient, love is kind."

I looked up the passage as soon as I got home.

"Love is patient, love is kind. It does not envy, it does not boast, it is not proud. It does not dishonor others, it is not self-seeking, it is not easily angered, it keeps no record of wrongs. Love does not delight in evil but rejoices with the truth. It always protects, always trusts, always hopes, always perseveres. Love never fails" (1 Corinthians 13:4-8 NIV).

Here is the insight I gleaned from this passage:

- *Be patient.* I'm sure there will be lots of times when I'll want to snap at him, but there's a better way.

- *Be nice.* I can do that. It's not difficult to be kind to the husband who has been kind to me for forty years. But it will be even more important to be nice if the time comes when he no longer knows how to reciprocate.

- *Don't envy.* It would be easy to envy others who don't have this cross to bear.

- *Don't get puffed up.* My bragging rights are nil. Without the Lord to see me through and the support of family and friends, I would be a basket case.

- *Do not dishonor him.* I will treat my husband with respect and build him up every way I can.

- *This is not about me.* It is about pouring myself into my husband's life and not seeking accolades. I already know there is great satisfaction in giving to others without expecting anything in return.

- *Do not be easily angered.* With God's grace, I will think before I speak and respond in kindness. If the situation is ugly and kindness doesn't work to calm the atmosphere, I can go to another room and take deep breaths to guard my own peace. Someone once said that the person who acts the ugliest needs love the most.

- *Do not keep a list of faults or grievances.* I will forgive quickly and thoroughly, leaving nothing behind to fester. This is how Drew and I have always resolved our problems, and I will continue to practice this habit.

- *Do not delight in evil.* This disease is devastating enough. There's no room for revenge or paybacks for any cruel things he might say or do as his mental capacities decline.

- *Rejoice in the truth.* I married a wonderful man who has been my steadfast defender, provider, protector, and friend. And the truth is, he will always be precious to me and his children and grandchildren.

- *Protect my husband.* As the days unfold before me, I'll be called upon to make many decisions—some big, some small—and I am committed to making them all with his best interests in mind, not for my comfort or convenience.

- *Trust God.* In trusting God, I can trust myself to discern whom else I should trust and turn to for advice as I find my way along.

- *Do not lose hope.* Regardless of how things appear, I hold onto the hope of knowing that God honors and rewards hidden acts of love.

- *Persevere.* I can only imagine how many times I'll want to throw in the towel as the disease advances, but love sees things through to the finish line. Lord, help me to have the staying power I need and a good attitude to go with it. I realize You are not pleased with those who shrink back.

- *Love never fails.* Because I anticipate faltering and making mistakes in my attempts to navigate unknown territory with Alzheimer's in our home, it's good to remember that God is love, and love never fails.

I realize these are lofty goals, but spelling them out and keeping them front and center from the very beginning certainly establishes a hopeful tone. Only time will tell how closely I come to keeping them.

April 11, 2014

The next morning, Drew and I began searching together through a mountain of paperwork on his desk to find any bills that hadn't been paid. I brought the big stack to the kitchen table and sorted them by their due dates. With him looking on, I wrote checks and put them in the envelopes. His job was to affix the return address stickers and stamps. I was struck by how slowly he moved and how long it took him to do this simple task.

When we finished, Drew took me to IHOP for a late breakfast. There I sat at the table, trying to muster enough energy to hold a coffee cup that suddenly held the weight of the world. Drew sat across from me, looking as carefree as a boy about to visit a toy store. With a contented smile, he raised his forkful of pancakes dripping with syrup and announced, "I love my life."

I mustered a convincing smile and thought, *Of course you do.* As his life became more simplified by the minute, mine was caving in on me.

May 11, 2014

On Mother's Day in 2014, Drew and I went for a long drive in search of where I lived as a child on Clayton-Dulaney Road, way off the beaten path, between Delaware and Maryland. Although the house that used to have rose arbors had been torn down and rebuilt, and the strawberry patches, fields of corn, and a mini-orchard of apple and pear trees were all overgrown, the surrounding area and roads hadn't changed. It was a beautiful day with lush greenery everywhere. As we drove, we talked heart-to-heart about our dads and their work, things our parents said and did, favorite Christmas toys, bike rides, and lemonade stands— things we had never discussed before. Just being in the vicinity triggered memories like Mom chasing my naked brother, Mike, around the yard with a garden hose because he had painted himself in poop.

Old memories suddenly seemed new to Drew as if he recalled them for the first time. That day, it was as though he saw *me* again for the first time.

It was like that balmy evening in May of 1975, when his Aunt Fannie (my daughter's babysitter) walked me across the street from her house to his and in the back door. "I brought you somebody," Fannie said (as if I were a gift). And the first words out of Drew's mouth were, "You sure brought me a pretty one." I let myself go there and saw him for the first time all over again, too.

And so, that Mother's Day of 2014, we began our second courtship—with a bank of thirty-nine wonderful years to draw on. We basked in it and gazed deep into each other's eyes, giving one another special little winks at Twin Trees Restaurant.

This "love fest" continued for a full week.

May 20, 2014

On a Tuesday night, as executive director of Mothers With a Mission, I dressed to attend a reception hosted by a non-profit organization for other non-profits. Drew sat in the bedroom watching television, and the smell of my perfume must have catapulted him back to the days when his first wife cheated on him. He demanded to know where I was going without him.

Even when Karen, our fund-raiser, came by to go with me, he crossed his arms over his chest and wouldn't hug me goodbye.

With his flawed memory, I thought for sure he would forget by the time I got home, but the suspicion only accelerated while I was gone. I reminded him that in all the years we'd been married, I had never given him a reason to doubt me. My words just bounced off him.

"I'm your faithful wife," I said.

"I've heard that before," he yelled.

This was a good clue. The jealousy had a root, and it made sense. His first wife left him for another man.

"I'm Candy, not Catherine," I said.

But his demeanor stayed the same. With his chin in the air, eyes narrowed, and a disbelieving smirk on his face, he grilled me about the event and who the people were.

The invitation that had come a month ago was addressed to me as the director of our non-profit organization, and I was allowed to bring one guest.

"Why didn't you ask *me* to go with you?" he asked.

"I did. I asked you *first* to be my guest, but you told me, 'You know how I hate those stand-around-and-talk-about-nothing things. Why don't you ask one of your girlfriends?'"

I saw a flicker of truth register in his eyes—and then pain, followed by remorse. He fell all over himself apologizing. "I don't know what came over me," he said. "I'm so, so sorry, so sincerely sorry."

In the midst of my hugging and kissing him and saying, "It's okay," he said, "I promise you that you'll never see that side of me again."

Of course, I know that it could happen again. If and when it does, I will cling to the knowledge that the real Drew is my protector and defender who would never intentionally give me even a moment's grief—certainly not jealousy.

May 25, 2014

I tried once, and only once, to talk to Drew about his condition. "Your memory isn't working like it's supposed to."

Those few words put panic on his face. "What? Are you saying there's something wrong with my brain?" His hands trembled and flew immediately to his face.

If I didn't know better, I would have thought he'd just stared into the eyes of the Devil himself. His agitation was so great and startling that I immediately began backpedaling.

"Well," I said, "you had that brain tumor removed, you know, and I think it may have damaged your memory."

His eyes darted from side to side, and then he squeezed them shut in a long blink. "Well, other people my age can't remember things, either."

"That's true," I said and vowed that never again would I confront him about Alzheimer's. He was finding a way to cope, so I grabbed hold. "Yep, you know Aunt Addie lived to be 103, and she always said, 'Old age ain't for sissies.'"

Some people like to be involved in their diagnosis, but others can't handle it. For Drew, denial is a comfortable fit. Indeed, denial can be an effective tool.

May 27, 2014

Over the last couple of years, responding to a nudge from God, I began weaning myself away from some obligations and responsibilities, and now I would need to part with other roles:

- dropping out of singing in the choir (which I had done for thirty-five years);

- closing out my Mary Kay business;

- streamlining the Fruitbearer Women's Retreat that I hosted; and

- prying my fingers loose from other ministries like Mothers With a Mission and Delmarva Christian Writers' Fellowship.

Feeling unplugged from friendships and leadership roles, I prayed, "Lord, who am I without all the things I do?"

And I heard Him whisper a few words that put everything in perspective, "You are My child and wife to Drew. There is a time and a season for all things."

May 29, 2014

I'm doing most of the driving because Drew can't remember his way to the restaurants anywhere but in town. At first, I would pipe up, "You missed your turn," or "Don't you want to go over there?" But he took offense, and rightly so. After I had learned to stop offering "advice" and wait until he asked for it, my transition into the off-balance world of Alzheimer's became easier to navigate. Instead of pointing out that he just missed a turn, I bit my tongue and allowed him to feel the awkwardness of trying to find the way on his own. After enough wrong turns and embarrassment, he began asking me to drive.

I've found a number of methods to keep him calm and happy, the most effective being to keep things simple and not over-explain or give too many details. Now and then, we recapture the bliss of that loving emotional place we discovered on Mother's Day, and he says he enjoys having me chauffeur him around. His memory continues to deteriorate, but he explains it away, which makes him content.

I had a hard enough time facing the situation myself, but breaking the news to the family was especially difficult. It had to be done face-to-face. One at a time, I filled them in. All three of our children had noticed changes over the years, so it didn't come as a major shock. Dana, my stepdaughter, asked if she could meet us for dinner once a week to make sure she had some quality time with her dad. Troy, my stepson, threw himself into the task of sketching out plans so we could add a deck to the back of our house. My daughter, Kim, and her family gave us support through phone calls and offers to help mow the lawn. And our grandchildren made time in their busy schedules to drop by for visits.

When I broke the news to my brothers and their wives, the family support and prayer base broadened. I began to feel less like it was all up to me.

My brother, Mike, made a simple statement that has stayed with me: "Don't forget your sense of humor." Nothing seemed funny at the time, but those few words have served as permission to view things through a more lighthearted lens than I might have otherwise. Faced with added responsibilities and life-altering decisions, it took a while for me to see the humor in anything. Eventually, I began to recognize and appreciate the amusing side of caregiving. I'll share some of those things later.

But first, it was important for me to grasp and manage the serious side of caregiving.

June 4, 2014

I'm feeling particularly loved and secure today. Drew is happily running errands and humming little tunes, and it's a gorgeous June day. God's grace and the words of my sister-in-law that came through her e-mail are hugging me. Lots of publishing stuff to focus on today, and I'm taking time out to get my nails done. It is good to savor the happy days.

June 5, 2014

I thought yesterday was a particularly normal day until we were on the way to Fenwick Island for dinner. But then, the signs I'm becoming all too familiar with began again. Drew was gazing out of the passenger window and didn't recognize that Indian River High School was our grandson Trevor's school, and when we passed the Pyle Center, he had no recollection of the many, many Little League games we had enjoyed there. The rest of the evening was enjoyable, and then in gentle conversation on the way home, passing through Roxana, he said, "Dana just had one child, right?"

"Yep, she and Troy both had one," I said. "Dana had a girl, and Troy had a boy." And then I rambled on about them being born ten days apart in December.

A little time passed, and then he said, "What's Dana's daughter's name?"

The moment I said, "Natalie," he recognized it and then said, "But we don't see her very often, do we?" That gave him an excuse and made him breathe easier. Then he added, "She and Trevor are both twenty-five, right?" And, by George, he was right.

Speak kindly today.
When tomorrow comes,
you will be in better practice.

—Anonymous

CHAPTER FOUR

Dreaded Legal Stuff

June 6, 2014

My friend Margery wrote, "I know tomorrow, Saturday, is your birthday. Will Drew remember? My heart weeps for the sadness you must feel along with so many other emotions. I'm glad you have Buttercup to talk with and walk with, and I know God's sustaining love and spirit helps keep you on track."

I told her that Drew remembering my birthday is not a problem because I just keep telling him, "Tomorrow is my special day" and make suggestions about how I want us to spend it. Bless his heart, he went out and bought me a card all on his own, and it was a good one. Then he looked in his wallet and didn't like what he saw, so he told me to go ahead and write out a check to myself for $500 or $1,000, whichever I wanted. Very generous, don't you think? If only he had a clue about the bank balance.

Tonight we went to a little pub, and I pretended it was our first time there. He tells everyone we meet that we've been married "almost forty years." Although it will only be thirty-nine years on the 29th of this month and I've been correcting him, this is probably the last anniversary he's going to be aware of. Since I trust we'll hit that magic number of forty, I'm going to go ahead and agree with him from now on. "Almost forty" is exactly right.

It's a strange thing having one foot in reality and the other in a dream world where things are pleasantly vague. He still wants to be my protector and confidant, and I love being safe in his arms, so we do a lot of snuggling and talking about the "mean people" who used to make us miserable until we found each other.

Before going to dinner, we made an appearance at Kade and Saige's Little League games tonight and strolled from one ball field to the other hand-in-hand in the pleasant evening air. Tomorrow we'll relax around the house and find another romantic place to celebrate my birthday dinner, and the kids will stop by at some point during the weekend. I'm savoring this little oasis.

June 28, 2014

Drew seems to have leveled off. I'm getting used to the temperament swings and memory glitches. I'm also spending an inordinate amount of time trying to get the finances in a manageable condition. My publishing and writing have taken a hit as he continually interrupts my work time to "chat," asks me to go with him somewhere, or invites me to watch TV with him. A little attention seems to satisfy him, and then I can get back to the keyboard, but my focus and concentration are, well, hampered. I'm praying that God will help me redeem the time as I try very hard to keep my priorities in perspective.

We both have colds. The mucus in my head makes it hard to think, and my energy level is nil. It feels like I'm living in a jar of molasses. Even so, while inching along on everything that matters,

I'm still at peace. We take naps almost every day and are sleeping well, so that's helpful.

July 4, 2014

Drew's mother died in the '80s, but her birthday was the 4th of July, and I always think of her on Independence Day. I wonder what advice she might have offered and if she would be pleased with my best efforts to love her son under these trying circumstances.

Drew and I watched fireworks on TV, so my hopes of getting our legal matters finalized fizzled as quickly as the burning embers.

July 12, 2014

Other than the two-week summer cold that zapped me of all energy, I'm feeling strong in spirit. Every time I'm tempted to worry, the Lord is quick to whisper to me, "I've got this." Drew continues to be his gentle, lovable self, and I pray that he will remain that way for the duration. I'm spending more time with him, appreciating each day, and he delights in hearing the stories of our life together over and over again.

July 14, 2014

I joined a monthly Alzheimer's support group. One of the first things someone told me was, "Love whoever shows up," which has become an anchor for me since the perception of reality with an Alzheimer's patient is often a mystery.

How do you love someone who is unable to show love in return? I'm truly discovering that love means giving of yourself to someone else without expecting anything back. Of course, if it's reciprocated, all the better. Nevertheless, love begins with kindness. In a word, "Be nice." (All right, that's two words). Love is the

Golden Rule—doing unto others as you would have them do unto you. Love sets an example by caring, which involves anticipating the other person's need without having to be asked. Love looks for opportunities to say or do things that will build up and encourage. Sometimes, love doesn't have to say or do anything—just being with somebody is enough.

Just as my first Alzheimer's support group meeting was about to close, the lady who was leading it asked me, "Do you have your legal affairs in order?"

My coat suddenly felt heavy in my hand. "We've been talking about updating our wills for ten years, so I guess I'll need to see a lawyer after the neurologist makes a diagnosis."

The lady just about jumped out of her chair. "You can't wait till then," she said. "You need to take care of that *before* he's diagnosed."

I'm sure my eyes were as round as marbles. "You mean I need to get my legal affairs in order *now*, before our appointment with the neurologist?"

"Absolutely!" she fairly shouted, and everybody echoed agreement. "Attorneys have to make sure a person understands all ramifications before a document can be legally executed. You don't want to wait until your husband is declared mentally incompetent. And another thing." Her words came quickly. "As well as an updated will and advance health care directive, be sure you get a durable power of attorney to cover legal and financial decisions."

Before I could comprehend all the terms, she shocked me again. "This is urgent," she said with compassion in her eyes. "I'm giving you an assignment: make an appointment with your lawyer before next month's meeting, and bring us a full report."

I had barely come to grips with the reality of my husband's debilitating illness along with my need for a support group. Suddenly, my knees were weak from the urgency of taking the initiative for dreaded legal documents.

July 15, 2014

The assignment seemed overwhelming since Drew has always had an aversion to dealing with legal matters. Fortunately for me, however, it turned out that he initiated the subject himself. As I was mulling over how to bring the subject up to him about revising our wills, ironically, he showed me a clipping from the newspaper about the sad situation with Casey Kasem's estate.

The article ends with, "Most important, talk. Have open conversations in which everyone is present. You need to speak to your family when you are competent to discuss your wishes, and I prefer that everyone is in the room at the same time."

It was the perfect springboard for me to suggest that we get the three kids together for a family meeting. He wouldn't hear of it. He wanted the two of us to do this on our own. Immediately, he launched into a spiel about a complex wll instead of the typical surviving spouse and then children.

The more he tried to identify specific assets and properties, the more confused and agitated he got. "I know what I want in my head, but I can't figure out how to explain it," he said.

That afternoon, with my heart pounding, I arranged to meet my stepchildren Dana and Troy, at McDonald's, a place where we could talk openly. It was the first time in our marriage that I had done anything behind Drew's back, but I reminded myself that the goal was to keep us both from being anxious or overburdened.

Looking into Dana and Troy's faces and going over the symptoms their dad was exhibiting was heart-wrenching for all of us. When our conversation turned to the urgency of updating the will, they said they wanted my daughter included equally with them.

"She's more than a stepsister," Dana said. "She's family—"

Troy finished her sentence. "She's our *sister*. We love Kim."

This choked me up big time—not only to hear them express their affection for Kim and me but because it also relieved the pressure of how I should advise the lawyer to draw up the papers. Not "his" and "mine" but "ours."

When I got home, I approached Drew again. Immediately, he became fixated on something complicated instead of surviving spouse and then children.

When I suggested that Steve Ellis, our attorney, should be able to help us sort it out, he said, "I'm not sure he's the right one."

I could tell by his body language that his listening mode was shutting down—maybe turning off. If I had any chance of getting this done, I had to back off. Even with feeling the urgency to get the legal issues resolved, I could only tell Drew that I trusted him to do the right thing, hoping to make him feel he had control of his estate.

Realizing I had given him the freedom to do it himself, he softened and reassured me, "We'll work this out. I want to be sure you're taken care of."

At least we're heading in the right direction.

July 24, 2014

After days of persuasion, with Drew continually resisting, we met with our attorney, Steve Ellis, on Monday the 21st to update our will and draw up a durable power of attorney. Within a few days, the documents were ready, so we went back to sit down with him and go over them.

Steve had barely begun explaining the first couple of paragraphs when Drew stood up and said, "This is too important to rush through. I have to take this home and study it."

We went home, and he began dissecting every line of legalese that, of course, only made him more agitated than before.

Drew fretted. "What if you remarry and some guy tricks you into signing over all your money to him? How can I be sure everything I own won't wind up in his hands?"

My assurances of guarding his assets for the children fell on deaf ears. No matter what answers I gave to his many questions, he grunted in disapproval and moved on to the next, only to grunt again and then raise his voice.

I have never been so frustrated in my life. If it hadn't been so urgent to get this done, I would have put it off for another ten years. I wanted to pull my hair out and scream because it seemed impossible to deal with the situation, but I knew better than to yell at Drew. I didn't want to risk the discord escalating to a higher level that could become our "new normal."

My frustration was through the roof. I couldn't help Drew understand that I was not trying to pull something over on him. Fear was present as well, whispering, *He's never going to let you finalize this will.*

After I'd said all I could yet nothing convinced him, I went outside and had a meltdown on the unfinished deck where I sat and sobbed to God, "I see no way out of this. He won't budge. I can't handle this. I don't know what to do."

His answer came as a whisper in my mind. *Call Dana.*

Dana has always been her daddy's girl, and he listens to her. I dialed her number and whimpered into the phone, "I need you." She was at the grocery store but said she'd come as quickly as she could.

My mind flashed back to when she was seventeen and said those same words to me, "I need you." She'd been dropping hints about wanting a Siberian Husky puppy, but Drew wouldn't hear of it. Still, she did her research in *The Guide*, found one in Hartly, Delaware, got $100 out of her savings account, drove over to see the blue-eyed ball of fluff, and wound up buying him on the spot. She named him Wolf. Telling herself that as soon as her dad saw the adorable puppy, he would cave in and let her keep it, she drove immediately to where he worked.

But Drew said, "No. I told you no, and I meant it. No more dogs. Take that puppy back to wherever you found it."

She couldn't bring herself to tell him that she'd bought it. Instead, she called me weeping so hard she could barely talk but somehow poured out the whole story. "Candy," she said, "I need you. I need you to convince Dad to let me keep him."

It was a bonding moment for stepmother and stepdaughter, which was the argument I used to convince Drew to let Dana keep Wolf (who was with us for eleven years).

This time, I was the one in need of an ally to convince Drew. Ten minutes passed since I made the call. At last, Dana breezed through the front door. I flopped into her arms like a wounded puppy. She ushered me with my red eyes and Drew with his tight expression into the kitchen where we examined the will together. She went through the paragraphs methodically, trying to comprehend them quickly and explain them to her father.

"Nobody's trying to trick you, Dad."

Troy came over and joined in, but Drew continued to rant and repeat his concerns. Still in output mode, he was unable to hear their rationale any more than he could hear mine. At least the tone of the conversation had calmed down a bit.

At last, Dana said something that brought closure. "The bottom line is this: I'm named as the executrix if something happens to Candy. She and I agree that however you want your assets handled, that's what we will do."

"That's right," Troy chimed in. "We're family, and we want you to be proud of how we handle things if you're not here."

Things were not resolved, by any means, but I was so exhausted that I turned to sleep as an escape.

July 30, 2014

The legal papers still on our kitchen table are the topic of conversation all day, every day. I need to get this finalized so I can breathe easier. The stress level for both of us is through the roof. So much for maintaining peace in our home. If only I didn't have to do the hard, necessary things. But I do. And I will.

August 3, 2014

I spent the weekend at the Greater Philadelphia Writer's Conference, where I fell into Nancy Rue's arms the minute I saw her. I cried on her shoulder, and she consoled me as only someone who has been my writing mentor and confidant for years could do.

Family members took turns checking on Drew, and he did well without me. When I got home, I learned that the only incident seemed to be a lost loaf of bread they searched in vain to find. It turned out the receipt showed he hadn't bought it after all.

We methodically went through the legal documents, and he seemed to be content. So I made "practice copies" of everything and had him sign and date them in preparation for our follow-up visit with the attorney on Tuesday. It was a wise move. Seeing his handwriting served as a concrete reminder to him that he had agreed to it while he questioned what we were doing another ten times.

August 4, 2014

We're back in uncertainty again this morning about the will. Yesterday Drew had everything clear, but today he woke up fixated on it and stuck on rehashing the same old things he still can't articulate. Even seeing his signature doesn't help today.

I have so much work to catch up on and so many details to attend to, but he wants me to sit with him while he reads and rereads the pages with worsening comprehension. And the minutes and hours are wasting away.

As I was dissecting the paragraphs for the hundredth time, he called me "ungrateful," which cut me to the core. I sobbed off and on for hours. My tears were probably as much about my grief over losing him as they were about the week-long frustration over the will and his ugly words.

The Lord has seen fit to put us through this, and He will strengthen me for the duration. Jesus once told His disciples, "Peace I leave with you; my peace I give you" (John 14:27 NIV). As long as I can guard my peace and remember who Drew truly is, I'll be fine. Prayers are essential, but I have to be careful whom I share my concerns with because he is in denial about anything being wrong with him.

August 5, 2014

Drew pouted, fussed, and fidgeted, right up until time to leave the house for our appointment with Steve Ellis.

"I'm leaving now, hon," I said with a smile. "It would be best if you went with me."

So he did.

No sooner had we greeted Steve, taken our seats at the well-polished mahogany table, and gotten through the first page to the signature line when Drew said, "I don't have to sign this. I need to take it home and study it."

Steve surprised us both when he said, "We did that once, and we're not doing it again. Drew, you *do* need to sign this."

Drew's voice raised a notch. "I don't have to sign *anything*, and you can't make me."

While my heart began to race, Steve remained calm and spoke in a low, friendly tone. "That's right," he said. "I can't make you sign anything." Then he reminded Drew how many decades he has done legal work for our family and asked if Drew still trusted him.

When Drew nodded, Steve continued with authority. "Well, let me explain how things will play out if you don't sign these papers.

He went through a lengthy explanation of how cumbersome it would be for his family to handle the assets he had spent a lifetime accumulating and how difficult it would be to make wise medical decisions on his behalf if he didn't have an updated will, POA, and advance health care directive. "Is that what you want?"

"Where do I sign?" Drew said.

We walked out of the office with executed documents in my hand and relief in my heart. *Thank You, Lord!*

August 10, 2014

I see changes in Drew every week, but he's still his gentle self. I'm learning which topics trigger anxiety and how to avoid them. But just when I figure something out, the next week I have to develop a *new* strategy because the old one didn't work as I expected. I feel off balance but need to be on my toes every day, nonstop.

When does a caretaker get to breathe? My dear friend Margery Mayer sends an e-mail now and then with this instruction, "Breathing in, breathing out," and that helps.

Now that Drew isn't busy paying bills and handling the rental properties, he has a lot of time on his hands and can't understand why I can't be his constant playmate. I would love to drop everything and play; but, of course, duty calls, and somebody has to be responsible.

All of this could be maddening, but I have dear friends who pray for me and send encouraging e-mails on a regular basis. Margery also passed this poem along, and it came at the perfect time because I've been grappling with ways to develop a mindset that will sustain me through the long and lonely journey ahead:

"Love's Lantern"
by
Joyce Kilmer

Because the road was steep and long
And through a dark and lonely land,
God set upon my lips a song
And put a lantern in my hand.

Through miles on weary miles of night
That stretch relentless in my way
My lantern burns serene and white,
An unexhausted cup of day.

O golden lights and lights like wine,
How dim your boasted splendors are.
Behold this little lamp of mine;
It is more star-like than a star.

*Every survival kit
should include a sense of humor.*

— Sol Luckman

CHAPTER FIVE

Bermuda Cruise

January 12, 2015

The balance of 2014 contained one situation after another, so I could no longer ignore or explain away the memory issues. Having watched my friend Wilma care for her husband at home, I prayed that Drew, like Elton, would retain his gentle disposition and not engage in combative behavior since it's my full intention to keep him here in the home he loves for the duration.

This time, when we met with Dr. Sugarman, I asked for a referral to a neurosurgeon. He recommended someone in the same practice, and I called Dr. Edelsohn's office that afternoon. The next available appointment was April 23rd.

April 2015

My goals from the beginning, and to this day, have been threefold:

1. To guard Drew's peace.
2. To honor his integrity.
3. To keep him happy.

In short, my desire is to maintain a sense of contentment in our home and be aware that God controls the events of each day.

Drew finds comfort in denial. I respect that. For him, denial is a helpful coping tool. I, on the other hand, am a realist who finds it easier to face the difficult things of life head-on by being well informed than by avoiding them. For me, ignorance is not bliss.

I missed a lot of clues in the beginning because I simply didn't know to look for them.

For years, Drew used to meet early every morning with a group of guys at McDonald's to solve the world's problems over steaming cups of coffee. About the time I retired from my full-time job, he began skipping their coffee klatch occasionally, and then he missed a whole week. When I asked about it, he said, "What man in his right mind wouldn't rather be here with you than being with a bunch of old guys?"

I felt flattered, and another clue went overlooked. Looking back, I wonder if he could no longer hold his own in conversation, even that long ago. Maybe it wasn't fun anymore and easier to avoid his friends than to risk being embarrassed.

April 23, 2015

The appointment with Dr. Edelsohn was tough on Drew. He didn't know the answers to simple questions and felt like he was being tricked. At the end of the session, Dr. Edelsohn said, "I've looked at your MRI, and can see that the brain tumor did do some damage. I'm sorry to have to tell you this, but I do see some signs of Alzheimer's." Drew just nodded his head as if he understood, but none of this registered with him. I, on the other hand, choked back tears to hear the dreaded word. This was a reality that would alter our lives forever.

When we got in the car, Drew was all smiles and said, "That went well, right?" Then he looked into my watery eyes. "What's wrong? Did I do something wrong?"

"No, honey," I said. "You did great. And I'm just fine. It was a good appointment. You don't have anything to worry about."

I filled the prescription for Aricept as soon as we got back to Georgetown and started him on it that night.

June 19-26, 2015

My family and I lived in Bermuda during my teen years. So, one of my heart's desires has been to take our whole Abbott family on a cruise together so I could share the beauty of the island with them. In light of Drew's some-sort-of-dementia, I figured it was now or never. I began exchanging e-mails and making plans as well as getting our passports in order. When the time came, eight of us booked cabins on the *Grandeur of the Sea*: Dana and her husband John, our grandson Trevor and his fiancé Jill, our granddaughter Natalie, her sister-in-law Alisa, and Drew and me.

I reserved Thursday for packing, but Drew was suddenly very needy, coming up with things to divert my attention all day. So I didn't begin to put any clothes in his suitcase until 9:00 p.m. When I turned my back to get something from his closet, he stuffed it all back in his drawers—a little here, a little there—so I had to search for everything like an Easter egg hunt. By the time I got his things where they belonged and zipped up his suitcase, it was 11:30, and I was too tired to even think of packing my own. So, I set the alarm for 4:30 a.m., which I figured would give me just the quiet time I needed to get my week's worth of clothes together in time to be ready for the limo van at 6:30. Before dozing off, I thought about that scene in the movie *Home Alone* in which the family oversleeps on the day of their big trip.

And sure enough, my alarm didn't go off. (I must have set it for p.m. instead of a.m.) At 6:15 I woke up to go to the bathroom and glanced at the clock, ripped my CPAP gear off my face and hollered, "Get up, get up! The driver will be here in fifteen minutes!"

Sure enough, the driver was on time, and I had just begun to pack. I met him at the door in my PJs, and he went and picked up Dana and John while I sped around the house.

Trevor and Jill arrived and put the luggage tags on for me while I tried to get my brain to work.

Drew helped by standing in front of me each time I turned around and finally saying, "I think I'd better get out of your way," which really did help.

Somehow (duh, the grace of God?), I got my act together by 6:45, and we drove off to pick up granddaughter Natalie and her sister-in-law, Alisa.

Drew sulked the minute we got in the van, complaining because the three girls kept talking and laughing. (Hey, isn't that what you're supposed to do when you're embarking on a tropical cruise?) He kept a steady monolog going: "It's too hot." "It's too cold." "It's too loud." "How long until we get back home?" Yep, he began asking when we would be going home as soon as we left Milford, and several times daily afterward, including the day we set foot on the island.

The weather was glorious, and everyone boarding the ship seemed to be in high spirits—except Drew. As we walked up the plank with the happy vacationers, Drew said louder than I would have liked, "I don't know how I let you talk me into this."

I flashed an apologetic look at the couple behind us.

And then he added, "You'll never get me on one of these things again."

On deck, Drew was perpetually grumpy. My mind was preoccupied with trying to figure out a way to relax and enjoy myself while keeping him entertained since he didn't want to participate in any of the activities the cruise line had to offer. While the others lounged at the pool on the 8th deck, Drew and I strolled around and tried out one deck chair after another. Dining was the one thing he looked forward to, so we ate our way to Bermuda.

As the ship neared the island on Sunday afternoon, Drew sat in a deck chair. I stood by the open window on the top deck and drank in the sight of the white-roofed houses. Fingers of sprawling greenery on the island stretched into the sapphire water that turned to shades of teal, turquoise, and aqua the closer we got to the Royal Navy Dockyards (which used to be the Navy base when I lived there).

At last, I was "home." We stepped off the ship from air-conditioned comfort into sweltering, humid air that smacked us in the face like the slobbery tongue of an oversized bloodhound. So much for the refreshing island breeze that I remembered.

Dana stayed with us while the younger generation scooted off to Horseshoe Bay, and John rented a pedal bike to explore on his own. Dana, Drew, and I walked around to get our bearings, shopped for gifts and the shampoo and conditioner I had forgotten to pack, and bought a two-day pass for unlimited bus and ferry service. We had an appetizer and beverages at an island bar/restaurant, where the service was as warm and friendly as I remember it, and the food was great. (It's rare to see Wahoo bites on a menu.)

Drew was anxious to get back to the ship for dinner at 7:00, and he wasn't interested in going back out that night. I guess our cabin felt safe and secure to him. So I contented myself with sitting on our stateroom balcony, overlooking the people below who were partying on the dock. At least the calypso music that wafted up brought with it a sweet wave of nostalgia.

I closed my eyes and felt myself drifting back to when I was young and the steel drums were a regular part of my life. Those were the "Do the Limbo" days when I enjoyed family beach parties at dusk with fish from the grill and fried bananas.

As I sat in the deck chair looking through the sliding glass door at Drew, who was hugging the covers in bed, I allowed myself to get excited about our beach outing the next day. But then a pang of misgiving hit me. How would he handle our first full day on the island? I brushed the anxiety away and concentrated instead on fond memories.

During my teenage years living there, John Smith's Bay was within walking distance of our home on the South Shore. Mom, my brothers, and I spent a lot of time there, soaking up the sun on the pink sand and splashing in the turquoise water while Dad was at work. I can still smell the scent of Coppertone suntan lotion, feel the salt water drying on my bronzed skin, and taste the peanut butter and jelly sandwiches and Keebler Pecan Sandies cookies warmed by the sun.

The next morning, I was up bright and early so I could squeeze into the miniature bathroom before Drew got up. When I came out, there he was, fully dressed in yesterday's clothes.

"But today is our beach day," I reminded him. "See, I have your bathing suit and shirt all laid out for you, right here."

He hadn't noticed. "This'll be fine," he insisted.

"No, honey, you have to put your trunks on. I need you to be able to go in the water with me."

"I don't need to go in the water."

Rather than insist, I told him that the whole trip was meant to be a special celebration of our fortieth anniversary. "I've been squirreling money away for ten years for this trip, and today's beach day with our family is the high point for me—something I've been dreaming of all this time." I went on and on, making every persuasive point I could think of, ending with, "So, can you please put your trunks on so you can enjoy it with me?"

"You saved for ten years for this trip?"

At least he got something out of my spiel. "Yes, I did. So, will you put on your bathing suit?"

"Sure," he said. "I always want to do whatever makes you happy."

I put his trunks in his hand, gave him a big hug, and went back into the bathroom for a couple of minutes. When I came out, there he was, putting his trunks over his Fruit of the Loom briefs.

"Oh, honey, no! You need to take off your underwear."

"No, I don't. I *neeeed* my underwear."

I had a quick, silent talk with myself and decided some battles weren't worth fighting. "Okay. Sure, you can keep your underwear on, but promise me you won't be a spoilsport."

"Okay," he said. "I'll be good."

From that moment on, he didn't whine or puff up like an inflatable toad. In fact, he looked relaxed and even joked around a little—even when he and I, along with Dana, Trevor, Jill, Natalie, and Alisa took the ferry to Hamilton and then had to trudge up steep sidewalks until we reached the central bus station. He didn't fuss when we piled into the bus and asked the driver to drop us off at John Smith's Bay. So, I began to allow myself to anticipate a stress-free day.

My heart soared as I gazed at "my" beach. It was exactly as I remembered. But, before we had a chance to put our toes in the pristine pink sand, Drew piped up, "I have to go to the bathroom."

"Sorry, hon. There are no bathrooms here. You'll just have to pee in the water."

He frowned and gave me a stern look. "I can't pee in the water. I have my underwear on!"

So much for my stress-free day. "Well," I said, "when we were here fourteen years ago, there was a porta potty over there." I pointed to the coral reef. "You stay here with Dana, and I'll go take a look."

I took off my shoes and traipsed through the sand, over prickly dried seaweed, and around the corner of the reef. It felt good to be alone for a minute, even if I *was* still on duty as a caregiver.

No porta potty.

I turned around to go back and tell him the bad news, and I almost bumped into him. He had followed me the entire way. "Oh! Well, as you can see there's no porta potty, so let's go ahead and get in the water."

"No," he said. "I need to take my underwear off. No one will see."

"You can't take your underwear off out here in the open." I turned my back to him and pointed in the other direction. "See? On the other side of that hill, there's a road up there with cars. People can look down and see you."

"No, they won't," he said calmly. "I'll be quick about it."

By the time I swiveled around, he was already bent over with his trunks and underwear pulled down to his ankles.

"No! You pull those up right now!"

"It'll be fine," he said, continuing to struggle. "You just stand there and block me."

So I did as I was told. I turned my back to him and tried to position the widest part of myself in front of his bare behind. Looking up at the traffic going by, I'm thinking, *Oh, yeah. We're going to be arrested for indecent exposure on our first day on the island.* But then I figured it would be okay. After all, drivers most likely weren't looking in our direction.

Just then, he yelled, "I'm going to fall!"

So, with visions of him gashing his head on the coral, I instinctively reached both hands behind me and grabbed his butt cheeks. "There," I said. "I've got you. It's okay."

It wasn't okay.

Right about then, two ladies on mopeds were driving down a dirt path from the road and then parked eight to ten yards away from us. There I stood, in front of Drew with my hands behind my back, watching them as they got off their bikes and took off their helmets. They were facing the other direction, and one of them walked away from us and toward the water.

I held my breath, silently coaxing the other woman to do the same. *If we're quiet, she won't know we're here.*

No sooner did the thought pass through my mind when Drew shouted, "It's stuck. I can't get it off my foot!"

The lady spun around and glanced our way. She did a classic double-take and stared at me long and hard with the strangest look on her face.

I couldn't let go of Drew's hiney or he would fall, and I didn't want him to know she was there. So I gave her a strange look in return, tilted my head, and lifted my shoulders in a "You-caught-us-and-I-don't-know-how-to-get-out-of-this" shrug.

She shook her head and left (no doubt to tell her friend about the strange sight she'd witnessed).

At last, I felt the waistband of Drew's trunks touch my fingertips, so I grabbed it and hoisted it the rest of the way up. We exhaled and walked back to join the rest of the family, who must have been wondering what had become of us.

Drew headed straight into the water to pee.

I headed to the beach blanket to tuck his underwear into our beach bag. I leaned over and whispered to Trevor and Jill, "Have I got a story for you," and headed into the water myself.

Oh, how refreshing that water felt. It only took a minute for the chill to wear off, and then it felt like bath water. I floated over to Drew, and we bobbed together for a few minutes until he left to sit with Dana in the shade. Trevor and Jill joined me among the aqua waves to hear "the rest of the story," and went back to their blanket laughing. Little by little, the others took turns visiting the ocean pool to hear my tale, which seemed to get funnier each time I told it.

I stayed in the water for more than an hour. After that, the plan was to go to Devil's Hole (where we could dangle a hunk of meat on a rope for tortoises to eat) and the Flatts (known for some cute little tourist shops I remembered from my youth). The lifeguard said we could catch a bus up the hill. "Just a five-minute walk," he said.

These were my old stomping grounds. My brothers and I used to ride our bikes up the same hill that the seven of us now trudged up, single file. We walked for about twenty minutes in the blazing heat to the Flatts, up and around one bend after another. I huffed and puffed, feeling that my face was beet-red—and not from the sun. Drew stayed close by me, and Jill, a nurse, stayed close by to check on us. So much for my stress-free day.

At last, we came to a deli where we bought bottled water and decided we were all too tired and hungry to go into the aquarium across the street. That's when I found out that Devil's Hole and the little shops had closed years before.

We waited in the heat for a bus with "Hamilton" in the destination window. Finally, here it came—but there it went, sailing right on by with a whole load of people inside. The next Hamilton bus was pretty full, too, but the driver stopped and allowed all seven of us to pile in and stand in the aisle. So, there I was—all two hundred pounds of me—weak-kneed from the day, holding onto a dangling strap as the bus heaved us left and right while the driver navigated the hills, dips, and curves of the island, not to mention the jolts at every stop and start. I used muscles I haven't thought about since we went snow skiing thirty years ago.

True to his promise to "be good," Drew never complained. Not once.

We made it safely back to the bus depot and walked downhill (praise the Lord) to find someplace to eat. The four twenty-five-year-olds chose the restaurant that only had seating on the second floor, so I got another workout going up the steep stairs. However, the spinach/cauliflower soup was worth the effort.

On Tuesday, our last day on the island, Drew and I were alone because Dana, John, and the kids wanted to do other things. We took a ferry from the Somerset dockyard to Hamilton and sat in a park for a while. Then we hailed a taxi and asked the driver to take us to Clearwater Beach where I used to attend beach parties and dances. The pavilion is called Gumby's (pronounced Gumbay's with the accent on the second syllable). Although it is now a bar, the gazebo where my classmates and I used to dance to vinyl records looked pretty much the same as it did in the early '60s. I recognized what had to be the original pay phone, and the coral bathrooms with rickety wooden doors on the stalls were *exactly* the same as I remembered them.

The locals at Gumby's told us that Cooper's Island, an area always gated off as a private community when I lived there, is now open to the public—with a small hidden beach just big enough for two. As we headed up the path to Cooper's Island, the Bermudian called out, "You have to hold hands—it's a tradition," which made it extra special.

Hand-in-hand, I led the way up winding dirt paths sprinkled with rocks. The familiar musky scent of moss-covered coral and Bermuda grass combined with soft gusts of warm air made me giddy. When we reached the top of the hill, I could see the former Air Force base and my old high school. The view of the ocean was spectacular, and we kissed as the surf lapped against the coral. It was very hot (we heard the locals complaining all day), so we didn't stay long. But, without question, enjoying those private moments with Drew was the most satisfying and romantic part of the trip for me. When we got back to Gumby's, the locals said it was a tradition for us to kiss, so we obliged them.

"Now, that's what I'm talkin' about," the guy said, and they all applauded while I nursed bittersweet thoughts.

Drew was eager to get back on the ship, so we boarded hours before we set sail. He wasn't at all gripy because we were headed home, but I noticed over the next several days that he seemed a little more off-kilter than usual. He became confused, repeatedly referring to his dinner roll as a baked potato and trying to use toothpaste as shaving cream (twice). Also, he couldn't grasp the concept that we had to be on the water for two days before getting home.

Finally, we were back in the American waters and awoke to find that we were already docked in Baltimore. We went to the dining room for breakfast, and the host seated us at a table with six strangers. Drew didn't like it, no matter how pleasant they were. He pouted between bites. While I was in the middle of a happy conversation with a lady to my right, he touched my arm and said, "I need to go to the bathroom."

I nodded. "Okay, I'll go with you in a minute," and then I finished my conversation. When I turned back to him, he was gone. He hadn't waited for me. *He'll be fine*, I told myself and resumed eating my breakfast. For a brief moment, things seemed normal to me. And then reality smacked me across the face.

Things were not normal. *Smack.*

Things would never be normal. *Smack.*

If he doesn't know where the restroom is, he knows how to ask for help finding it. But, he'll never be able to find his way back to me with all these tables and people.

I could never let my guard down—not even for a minute.

I didn't know where he was. How many minutes had he been gone? Two and a half?

I put down my fork, grabbed my purse, and raced past the smiling stately waiters, through the glass doors, and into the lobby—only to find it packed with a huge crowd of disembarking passengers with suitcases.

What if he got in line with them and walked off the ship without me?

Frantically, I peered from left to right and back again as I worked my way to the other side of the lobby toward the restrooms. I didn't see him. What color shirt was he wearing? At last, the men's room door was directly in front of me. *Now what? I can't go in there.*

Suddenly, the maître d' of the restaurant stepped forward with concern in his face that reflected the *PANIC* in mine. "What can I do to help?"

"My husband has Alzheimer's, and I've lost him, but I'm hoping he's in here—in the men's room."

"Tell me his name. I can go in and call for him."

"Drew. His name is Drew."

He opened the door. "Mister Drew, are you in here?"

And then I heard the sweetest sound on earth. "Yes, I'm in here."

June 27-July 3, 2015

The first morning at home, lying in our bed when he woke up, Drew insisted we were still on the ship and wanted to know when we would be home.

It took him a full week to adjust. The trip was hard on him, which convinced me more than ever that I needed to keep him calm.

The trip was hard on me, too. What I thought would be a relaxing respite turned out to be another level of intensive caregiving. However, the weather was lovely, and the memories were nostalgic. In retrospect, I think the underwear story alone was worth it.

Kim stopped by one day. After she had left, Drew asked, "Who was that?"

Even talking about her growing up here or mentioning Wyatt and the kids didn't help. But he did ask me to make a copy of the picture that's on the refrigerator of the four of them and write their names down on it and how they're related.

So very sad. Yet the photograph and labels serve as a helpful aid for Drew to stay connected and content. The fact that he wanted to know who they are is a sweet comfort to me.

*Our temper is one of the few things
that improves the longer we keep it.*

—W. B. Knight

CHAPTER SIX
Nightmares and Suspicion

September 1, 2015

A charley horse woke me up abruptly, so I jumped out of bed and hobbled all around the bedroom and into the kitchen where I found Drew standing at the bar eating his cereal.

"I've got a bad cramp," I said, still prancing around. "How are you today?"

"Not good," he said.

"Not good? Why? What's wrong?" I asked, slowing my prance to a pace.

"You broke my heart."

"I what? Broke your heart? That's a bad joke." I slowed from pacing in circles and glanced up at him. His chin quivered, and his eyes brimmed with tears.

"You're serious. I thought you were kidding."

A tear rolled down his cheek. "Yes, I'm serious," he said. "Aren't you leaving me today?"

"Oh, honey. No way. Why would you say such a thing?"

"Because your suitcases are in the bedroom. Aren't you packing up and leaving today?"

"No way." I cupped his face in my hands. "Oh, honey. You had a bad dream—a nightmare. There are no suitcases in the bedroom, and I'm not going anywhere. This is my home. You are my life."

No matter what I said, he was convinced that I had said horrible things and was trying to backpedal but would still be leaving him soon.

"See?" I would say over and over again, "I'm right here, and I'm not going anywhere." My repeated vows of affirmation and love just bounced off him as if those words didn't count.

For three whole days, he badgered me about the imaginary cruel things I had said to him and how I was planning to leave. I assured him of my love and devotion every way I knew how, but every time I thought we had things resolved, he would bring it up again. By the time we went to bed that night, it felt like the ordeal might be over.

I awoke at midnight and reached over to pat him. When he asked what was wrong, I told him it was just a love pat, and he said, "Oh yeah, pat me while you can before it's too late."

"What do you mean by that?" I asked. When he answered with the same old broken record, I figured since I was wide awake, we might as well get into it.

Back and forth we went, with him saying his mind was crystal clear about my threat to leave, and me saying that I never did and only wanted to be with him and love him. He crossed his arms over his chest and gave me a hard stare.

When I told him in tears how much I needed him and cherished him, he said, "Why didn't you tell me that before?"

I usually try to guard myself against mentioning his short-term memory loss but couldn't help myself this time. "I *did* tell you those very words—several times a day for the past three days, but you don't remember." Well, you can imagine how that set him off.

"So, you're saying I made all this up and I don't remember? I remember all right." And then he launched into citing the words he believed I said.

"Sometimes I'll tell you what you want to hear," I said, "but not this. I'm not laying claim to any of the nonsense that happened in your bad dream." I sat in the chair next to the bed and looked into his eyes, and they were cold toward me. "How do we get past this and back to the real us?" I asked.

"I don't know," he said and seemed to soften. "Either my mind is going, or yours is. I'm beginning to worry about you."

I moved closer and took his hands. "Whether it's me or whether it's you doesn't matter. We're in this together, and we need a fresh start so we can put this behind us for real. Maybe we could try forgiveness."

His eyes showed a spark of interest.

"So," I said, "will you forgive me for anything I said or did that hurt you?"

"Yes," he said as he squeezed my hand. "I forgive you."

"And now it's my turn," I said. "I forgive you for . . ." I felt a chuckle bubbling up. "For having a bad dream." Never had laughter felt so good.

We both laughed until our sides hurt.

"Nonsense," he said. "That's exactly what this amounts to."

I breathed a sigh of relief. "Absolutely. Let's put this nonsense into a closet, lock the door, and never open it again."

September 2, 2015

This wasn't Drew's first horrendous nightmare. Shortly after he began taking Aricept, he had dreams that got progressively worse and more frequent. At first, they were about someone chasing him or experiencing a near miss with a vehicle, but then they turned dark like a series of horror movies that had him trapped. Some he remembered, while others were so horrific that he couldn't articulate them. And now this—being convinced that I'm leaving him.

So, I called Dr. Edelsohn and told him that the medicine seemed to be helping Drew with his cognition during the day, but I was concerned it could be causing his nightmares. He said that it absolutely could be the culprit and recommended that I give it to him in the morning instead of at bedtime like the instructions recommended.

Fingers crossed.

September 3, 2015

A nurse once told me that for male Alzheimer's patients, one of the last things to go is their interest in sex. I'm going to risk getting a little personal here because I think it's important to talk about this vital element of a healthy marriage. Now that we're in our golden years, admittedly our sexual activity has mellowed, but the winks, innuendos, and overall foreplay have become even more satisfying.

For example, the next night, I sensed Drew's temperament clouding over, again. He was sitting in his recliner in the bedroom, and I had just come out of the bathroom with just my nightie top. But instead of reaching for the bottoms, I picked up a toy to throw to Buttercup, our cocker spaniel. When I tossed it, I accidentally flipped up the hem of my pajama top and Drew laughed and applauded. "What did I just see?" he said. "Do it again."

And so, I did. Again and again, with Buttercup jumping and fetching, and Drew and I splitting our sides over this silly spur-of-the-moment peep show. The joy on his face was priceless—better than sex.

We both slept with smiles on our faces that night.

September 9, 2015

My friend Kathi called while I was driving, and I told her I'd call back as soon as I got home.

"You've been on my mind a lot lately," she said when we connected. "What takes you out driving at 8:30 in the morning?"

"I had to take Drew for his haircut because last time he couldn't remember where to go." Then I proceeded to fill her in on the latest challenges, like his increasing boredom if I'm not with him every minute.

"So what are you doing to take care of yourself?" she asked.

I had to stop and think. "Well, I have a corner in my office where I keep my Bible and devotional, and I try to find ten minutes of undisturbed time there every day. Oh yes, and I was able to get away with my stepdaughter to attend the Women of Faith conference last month. Ten thousand women praising God together truly built me up." I took a breath. "And before that, when I was about to lose it, I spent forty-five minutes alone in a parking lot next to a dumpster, crying and letting the Lord comfort me."

"Oh, Candy," she said. "I'm so sorry you have to go through this."

She asked whether family members or friends could stay with Drew for a short block of time on a regular basis so I could look forward to a time of solitude once a week. I told her they have offered, but Drew says he doesn't need a babysitter and becomes agitated if I even suggest someone might come by for a visit while I'm running errands.

"Here's where we are," I said. "He tells me he's fine by himself, but the truth is that he gets easily bored. He used to cut the grass, which gave me a nice block of time, but he doesn't want to do that anymore, so our grandson is helping with that. Besides, leaving the house for an hour or two for my benefit won't help me because I already don't have enough time to do everything since I'm responsible for all the bills and household responsibilities in addition to my own business."

Kathi sighed into the phone. "Candy," she said, "you need to realize it's not all about him. It's about your ability to handle this long term. If you keep putting him first and accommodating his every want, unsuspected resentment can build up, and you can burn out. It's time for you to put some safety valves in place. It's not good for either of you if he becomes lazy and doesn't do the things he can. So tell me, what can he do?"

"I guess it's not so much a matter of laziness as it is the need to be needed."

Instantly, I had a flashback to last winter when I broke my right wrist. For several months, Drew rose to the occasion by helping me get dressed and assisting with other things I couldn't do myself. He has always been my protector and hero. For a brief time, my broken wrist gave him back his self-respect because he had a purpose. I remember thinking that when my wrist healed and I regained my independence, I should be intentional about finding things he could do for me. I still hadn't done that.

Conviction pricked at my soul as I realized that subtly, over the last few months, I'd redoubled my resolve to handle everything—and handle it well. Now, faced with Kathi's question, "What can he do?" it was clear that I hadn't handled things well at all.

Still mentally sorting through all this, I answered her question. "He's good at cleaning if I point out an area that needs it, but I have to be prepared to answer a dozen questions about which products he should use." My mind raced to think of other things he does around the house. "He cleaned the toilet yesterday. And he empties the dishwasher, along with the washer and dryer. But he can't sort the clothes or figure out the buttons, so I can't just delegate the laundry to him. He's good about checking the doors every night several times to be sure they're locked."

As with children, Kathi pointed out, sometimes it's easier to do things ourselves—especially when they don't do it as we would like. However, there are more important things at stake than "doing it right" and efficiently.

She prayed with me over the phone for the Lord to provide godly wisdom and creativity so I can find refreshment for myself, as well as ways to guide Drew toward being more active and engaged in things he can do on his own.

As she prayed, the names and faces of several of my Christian sisters came to mind, and I knew I needed to reconnect with them because their presence always builds me up. As soon as I got off the phone, ideas began to flow about things I could ask Drew to do for me. The first one was to clean out the cupboards with the canned goods, most of which were well beyond their expiration dates.

I turned on Pandora radio in the kitchen to our favorite Letterman station and told him it was "mood music" for a sticky job I was about to ask him to do. He rolled up his sleeves and began tackling it immediately, with gusto. Even better, you know what he said as I was about to return to my office? "Have I told you lately how much I love you?"

Within half an hour, the sound of his voice wafted down the hallway. "Mrs. Abbott," he said with a mock British accent, "the butler pantry is ready for your first inspection."

By the time I got to the kitchen, his arms were elbow deep in suds in the sink, washing the rust off a Lazy Susan. "If you'll sort out the bad ones," he said, "I'll put the good stuff away."

While I was sorting the cans, he looked up and said, "This is not *work*, you know. It's what you do when you love somebody."

I'm banking this day as one I can draw on if and when the "bad dream" negativity strikes again.

September 10, 2015

In the wee hours of the very next morning, I reached over to pat Drew on the arm while he was sleeping, only to find out that he was wide awake and hadn't been asleep at all.

"Is everything all right between us?" His words made my heart sink.

My assurances began again in earnest, and I reminded him of the fun we'd had all day. He said he remembered, but I could tell he was still troubled.

One of our smoke detectors began signaling little sporadic beeps, so we figured we might as well change the battery. At 2:00 a.m., there we were with a step stool, taking turns trying to quiet the thing and get the cover back in place.

Returning to bed and still wide awake, we watched television for a while. Then, during a commercial, Drew said softly, "I think I have some kind of insecurity." I could tell he had something more to say, so I waited. "Maybe something to do with Catherine?" His first wife had left him for another man more than fifty years ago.

This makes sense. With Alzheimer's, the short-term memory (present) loses focus, but the long-term memory (past) becomes clearer.

We discussed it. "I think you've had a soul wound," I said and suggested we ask God for help in dealing with it. We joined hands, and I prayed that the Lord would heal the deep wound in his mind and emotions, take away his insecurities, and give him peace.

As soon as I finished praying, a Scripture popped into my mind about taking every thought captive. I jumped out of bed to look it up and found 2 Corinthians 10:5 (NIV): "We demolish arguments and every pretension that sets itself up against the knowledge of God, and we take captive every thought to make it obedient to Christ."

Drew seemed to understand but said he wanted to study it in the morning. And then he said, "It would help if you wrote a note that I could look at that says you love only me."

Whoa! Why didn't I think of that? A love note. Sometimes the basic childlike things are the most effective.

In the morning, I placed a note on the marker board on the kitchen table where he couldn't miss it: "I love you, and only you!" with a heart beneath it; then, I added, "Always and Forever."

If I ever need to go away overnight, I think I'll type it up in big, bold letters and plaster a dozen copies all over the house.

September 17, 2015

Drew cut a little grass with the push mower last night around six, and I sat on the deck waiting for him to finish. After he had taken his favorite shirt off and hung it on the back of one of the wicker chairs, I noticed how dirty the inside of his collar was. About the time I was making a mental note to include it in the laundry, he finished up and sat across from me under the umbrella.

Now, you need to know that Drew has a significant hearing loss caused by Meniere's disease, which brings an added layer of challenge to our conversations.

Since the shirt was on my mind, I mentioned how it needed to be washed.

"What?" he said.

I repeated myself.

"What is it we're supposed to watch?" he asked.

Sometimes it helps to rephrase things, so I told him that I noticed his shirt smelled musty when I hugged him that morning.

Again, he didn't understand.

"Your shirt stinks," I said, trying to be concise.

"So, you're saying I stink?"

"No, your shirt stinks. I think I need to do a load of laundry before we go to bed so you can have it in the morning."

We did three loads before going to sleep. I sorted the clothes, and he carried them to the washer and emptied the dryer for me. But I noticed he seemed distant, and his goodnight kiss was more of a peck than a real kiss.

"Sundowning," or Sundowner's Syndrome, is a form of confusion that may occur with various types of dementia, such as Alzheimer's disease, that begins late in the day and often carries into the night. I thought this might be what we were dealing with, so I chose to act as if everything was fine.

But his first words in the morning were, "Did you tell me I stink, or did I dream that?"

"No, I never said *you* stink, but I did say your shirt needed to be washed."

"You did, too. You looked at me and said, 'You stink.' Are you thinking of leaving me?"

I countered with my fullest recollection of yesterday's discussion and finally had to admit that I probably did say those very words. And then I explained it was only about the shirt, never about him— that I will love him always and forever and didn't understand why he kept going to a negative place in his mind. He seemed relieved, so I added, "Get happy!"

He looked at me and said, "Sh*t happens?"

I cracked up because he hardly ever swears. "Now, there you go," I said. "That's the perfect example of the difference in our attitudes. I say 'Get happy,' and you hear 'Sh*t happens.'"

"Yeah," he said. "Sometimes I misinterpret."

September 21, 2015

I took over the household finances a year ago, and I'm a little less tentative. I've learned how to embrace the challenge of bank accounts, rental properties, and bills that used to scare the pants off me. In the process, I've learned some things that work and some that don't.

My first task was to round up all the bits and pieces that Drew had strewn here and there and then put likes with likes. In the beginning, I paper-clipped batches together—electric bills, phone bills, insurance bills, and credit card bills—and sorted them by urgency. When I was steeling myself to do the hard things, I guess my facial expressions and body language sent Drew some negative signals, and he became agitated.

It took me a while to realize that even though he can't express himself like he used to, his emotional receptors are no less keen. Drew has always been tender and sensitive, qualities I have always loved about him. But with Alzheimer's, this can be a double-edged sword by which he easily takes offense. It's one thing to guard my tongue so I don't snap at him, but it's another to monitor the subtle signals I send.

At one point, I felt all alone in handling the finances, and then he complained that he didn't know what was going on. I wanted to scream that it was bad enough having to bear all the burden of it without explaining my every move to him, which was like doing it twice. But I caught myself in time, took a deep breath, and apologized for being so gung-ho that I left him out. I reminded myself that everybody needs to be needed and feel a sense of purpose.

Again, I had a flashback to December when I broke my wrist and promised myself when I got better that I would try to depend on him for things he could do for me I normally would do myself.

So, when I was ready to tackle the bills today, I told him I needed his help. I showed him the balances in the checkbooks, what bills needed to be paid, and their due dates. *Together*, we agreed on priorities, and we're now both at peace.

Together. There's magic in that word.

September 22, 2015

The good news is that Drew's nightmares have stopped, so switching his Aricept to the morning instead of the evening has solved that problem. Several friends recommended a supplement of turmeric/curcumin, so I've added that to his medication routine, and he seems a little more alert.

The bad news is . . . our dog is getting fat. Me, too. What I didn't see coming is that Drew would find purpose in feeding us— *all the time.*

"Are you hungry?" he says. My auto-pilot response is, "Sure." Now, I can't blame him for what I eat because the things that go into my mouth are up to me. But the truth is, I'm tired of dieting and denying myself the comfort foods that are always within arm's reach. I'm going to have to do something about this—by gathering some discipline and self-control from somewhere, especially since I'm a diabetic and need to guard my health.

But Buttercup, our cocker spaniel, doesn't have any desire for willpower. In fact, she has learned that if she stares at Drew long enough, he will feed her again, even if she has eaten twice in the last fifteen minutes. Initially, I would tell him she just ate, but he'd say things like, "I guess I can't do anything right," or "Why are you always fussing at me?" It's not uncommon for Buttercup (this is gross) to vomit a bowlful of half-digested food, which I used to show Drew, but it only made him feel bad. So now, I just clean it up before he sees it.

When the veterinarian scolded me for how much weight Buttercup had gained since her last checkup, I explained our circumstances and asked his advice.

"You're in a tough spot," he said. "But your number-one priority is your husband and his peace of mind. It's as much a matter of quality of life as anything. Buttercup won't live as long as she would if you monitored her diet, but she'll die happy."

Maybe if I throw her a ball, we'll both live longer.

But this is no trivial matter. I need to stay healthy so I can take care of Drew. I've heard from the beginning, "The caregiver needs to take care of herself." In my case, that means eating the right foods at the right times and moving more. How do I do that when my appetite is raging, and all I want is mashed potatoes and ice cream? Not to mention that my willpower is shot. I know that if I eat as I should, my cravings will fall in line—but I don't want to. It takes energy to think and plan.

Besides, I've had a cold for a week. I'm almost glad because it gives me an excuse to stop the world mentally and get off. Drew has been doing a good job of letting me sleep and feeding me chicken soup.

He's also feeding me a steady dose of affirmation, telling me much how much he loves me and marveling (several times a day) about how wonderful our forty years together have been. You can imagine how soothing those words are.

Last night, as we were getting ready for bed, he asked, "How many nights have we slept together?"

"Good question, hon." I grabbed a calculator and started punching buttons. "Not counting the three months since our anniversary, that would be 14,600 nights."

He gazed lovingly at me and said, "That's a lot of nights." And then he added, "Which side of the bed do I sleep on?"

At first I thought he was joking, but when he pulled back the covers on my side of the bed, and I looked into his eyes, I knew he truly didn't know.

Fortunately, about that time I sneezed and had to blow my nose, which gave me time to swallow the pain and come up with an answer.

"You usually sleep on that side of the bed," I pointed and winked. "But we could switch if you want. After all, variety in the bedroom is healthy for a marriage, you know."

*The greatest gift
you can give another
is the purity of your attention.*

— Richard Moss, author

CHAPTER SEVEN

Moon, Mosquitoes, Music, and My Heart

September 23, 2015

Tonight is the fourth in a series of "blood moons" (lunar eclipses during which the moon turns red). Drew and I stood on our deck looking up at a perfectly full moon. Although it would be another hour or so before the eclipse began, Drew insisted that we take a picture of it, but the view from our house wasn't satisfactory.

"Let's go out to the country club where we can see it better," he said.

"We can see it fine from here," I told him. But for him that wouldn't do, and he became agitated. On second thought, it's rare for him to make a suggestion to go anywhere, so I figured it was a good idea.

"Yes, let's!" I said with as much enthusiasm as I could muster.

I found his camera, we hopped into the car, and I began to drive. When we turned the corner by Delmarva Christian High School, I said, "This is a good spot. With that open field, we can pull into their parking lot and have a great view."

That didn't suit him. He had his mind set on the view from the golf course.

In another minute or so, as we approached Sussex Pines Country Club, we realized that the trees were now full grown. Since there was no "view," I kept driving. When we came to a V in the road, I asked him if I should go left or right.

"Right," he said, and almost immediately after I turned onto that road, there was the Georgetown Wastewater Reclamation Facility surrounded by wire fencing with an open view of the sky above the massive mound.

"There!" he said. "Pull into that gravel driveway."

No sooner had I parked than he got out with the camera. I was about to suggest he wait until the eclipse began, but he was already out of the car, leaving the passenger door open. I watched him fiddle with the camera for a couple of minutes and was thinking about getting out to help him figure out which button to push when a strange sort of movement caught my eye.

I blinked to clear my vision, but the cloud of tiny black dots was still there, getting thicker and thicker by the second around the dome light.

Mosquitoes! Hundreds of them. Attracted to the light, they were flitting and swarming in circles right in front of my face! I began swatting and batting at anything that looked like a button that might turn the light off when I realized *Drew's car door was wide open,* so it wasn't going to go off.

I called for Drew, but he couldn't hear me. Because I couldn't reach across the console, I thought about getting out so I could close his door. However, I didn't want to open my own door and let more in or walk out into the mother nest of them. While I was frantically trying to think about what to do first and how to get away from the mosquitoes, Drew s-l-o-w-l-y turned and started walking back to the car. He was looking down at the camera and didn't notice his panicky wife waving wildly at him.

"Quick! Get in and close your door!" I yelled. "We have to get out of here!"

He noticed the mosquitoes right away. "Drive fast. We'll roll all the windows down, and they'll fly out."

And they did. I drove with my left hand, shooed them out with my right, and we laughed all the way home.

Drew got into his PJs right away and settled in for the night. An hour later, I stood on the deck watching the eclipse make its way slowly over the smiling face of the moon. When it was at its peak, I invited Drew to join me, and we enjoyed the spectacle in peace.

And you know what? Baby mosquitoes don't bite, so our adventure didn't leave us itching.

September 25, 2015

"I know how to make some extra money," Drew said with a boyish grin as he came into my office. "Kisses, ten cents." And then he bent down and kissed me.

I giggled and hugged his neck. "You're not allowed to kiss anybody else, you know."

"Wouldn't think of it."

"So, I guess at ten cents a kiss, I'm going to go broke." I reached for my wallet.

He waved the wallet away and gazed at me over his shoulder as he left the room. I could tell that mentally he had a satisfied skip in his step from entertaining me.

There's a lot of little boy in my husband. His playfulness is one of the things I've loved about him from the start. At this stage of Alzheimer's, his childhood memories are becoming more vivid. Now and then, he'll break into song with "Happy Trails to You" or "Home on the Range" and tell me for the umpteenth time about Roy Rogers touching his hand while riding Trigger when his dad took him to Philadelphia as a child. We sang a little bit of "She'll Be Comin' 'Round the Mountain" together in the car yesterday. Funny, he's never been much of a singer until now.

Often it's the little things that make up the bulk of life, so it's wise to savor and reflect on them. As things progress (or rather decline) and the hard times come, I'm hoping that recording some of these "little things" will help me recapture the "real Drew" and bring me joy.

Studies have shown that music is a powerful aid to those with Alzheimer's. Right now, Drew is at his computer listening to "Only You" by the Platters on iTunes. He has it set to repeat, and I think we're on the tenth time if my count is correct. "Only You" is his favorite. Whenever he identifies a song he likes, I add it to his collection. So far, the ones he plays most often include,

"Crazy" by Patsy Cline

"Take My Breath Away" from the Top Gun soundtrack

"Have I Told You Lately" by Rod Stewart

"Only the Lonely" by Roy Orbison

"Oh, Love That Will Not Let Me Go," his favorite hymn

"Statue of a Fool" by Jack Green

"Love Story" by Andy Williams

"Somewhere Over the Rainbow" (the IZ version, by Isael Kamakawiwo'ole, not The Wizard of Oz)

"It's Magic" by Kidz Bop, the song from 1975 (the year we met) which we claimed as "our song."

I'm savoring these words of this quote by Arne Garborg: "To love someone is to know the song in their hearts and sing it to them when their memory fails."

October 4, 2015

Drew kept insisting that today was Saturday when it was really Sunday. Back and forth we went. "Today is Saturday, isn't it?" he'd ask, and I'd answer, "No, hon, today's Sunday." After the sixth time of this pleasant banter getting us absolutely nowhere, I said, "You know what? It doesn't matter whether it's Saturday or Sunday because I love you just the same."

And that was the end of that.

Well, I guess I can't take all the credit. Truth be told, he happened to find the newspaper at the same time and noticed that it said "Sunday" on the front page.

October 5, 2015

Things can turn on a dime. This time, it's about *my* health.

I had a routine appointment this afternoon with Dr. Palekar, my primary care physician, and I began to cry when I updated him about Drew's condition and the pressure I'm under to keep everything in balance while putting on my happy face. After supplying me with tissues, he told me what everybody else says: "You need to take care of yourself."

And then, he began my exam. The lab results were surprisingly normal in spite of my weight gain and high blood sugar readings. He told me to call my endocrinologist to see if my diabetes medicine needed to be adjusted, so I added that to my mental to-do list.

My blood pressure was 111/70, but my pulse was 141. He raised an eyebrow and got out his stethoscope to listen to my lungs and heart.

"You're really racing around in there," he said and then called for the nurse, who ran an EKG—twice. He studied the readout. "Your heart rate is 140, and it's continuous. It's like you're running a marathon day and night, even when you're sleeping."

"No wonder I feel tired and weepy," I said. "It's stress, right?"

"Stress is a factor, but it wouldn't cause the numbers to go higher than 100." After confirming with me that I didn't feel dizzy, short of breath, or have a headache, he added that I wasn't perspiring either. "If you were symptomatic, I would put you in the emergency room. Instead, let me call your cardiologist and see what he says."

Over the phone, the cardiologist and my primary care physician agreed that I had atrial flutter and advised doubling one of my medications. The cardiologist said he wanted to see me in his office the following day.

"Since your heart cath in May was clear, we think it's your electrical system," Dr. Palekar said. "If the change in medication doesn't work, the next step will be to shock your heart back into rhythm."

Whatever it takes, I thought. My heart was already breaking emotionally. Maybe at least they could fix it physically.

The next day, I e-mailed my writing buddies to pray for me. When one of them replied that it was stress-related, I was surprised at the words that flowed out of me in response: "The stress is behaving like grief, which it certainly is to a great extent. And grief charts its course, ebbing and flowing when we least expect it. I do need to get myself in a position to handle the long haul."

Then I made a call to a therapist to discuss my emotional and mental condition. We set up an appointment for Thursday in her office above the garage of her home.

October 6, 2015

"Your heart rate is in the danger zone," my cardiologist said. "You're going to need a cardioversion to shock your heart into rhythm."

Our grandson's wedding is in two weeks. "Can it wait?"

He looked startled. "You don't understand. This is urgent. Can you be at the hospital at 7:30 tomorrow morning?"

I had enough trouble comprehending this, but Drew couldn't understand it at all. Worry was plastered all over his face as he kept asking, "Everything's all right, isn't it?"

And I kept answering, "Everything's going to be fine." It's surprising how giving assurance to someone else can calm you down while everything in you is screaming, *No! It's not all right!*

As I fought to keep from crying, my own words echoed in my mind. *Everything's going to be fine.* Instantly, a strong sense of the Lord's presence swept over me, calming my fears. It was as if God has spoken those words to both of us.

Instead of panic, praise welled up inside of me. *Thank You, Lord.*

October 7, 2015

Bright and early, Dana arrived to drive us to the hospital. Since Kim was teaching, she kept in touch by phone and text. Our minister was already in the waiting room, and Troy came a little later. After the nurses had prepped me, we held hands and prayed.

The cardioversion on Wednesday took only one hour from the start of the procedure until they discharged me. I went to sleep the minute we got home and was still dizzy when I woke up. I thought the hardest part was getting over the effects of the anesthesia.

But that afternoon and later that evening, my body began to ache as if I had the worst flu ever. I could barely move. Drew hovered over me, offering chicken soup and a helping hand to get to and from the bathroom.

Somewhere in the midst of my pain and mental fog, I remembered to call my therapist and tell her I would have to reschedule. Just thinking about climbing the stairs to her office made me feel faint. Besides, I figured the reason I had been on the verge of tears wasn't so much Drew's situation but my heart problems. Yeah, when it came time to talk to a professional, I needed to have my ticker behaving so my head could be clear.

By Friday morning, my diaphragm was so tight I could barely breathe. Because I was scheduled to take the minutes at a family meeting, I called Kelly, my sister-in-law, to tell her I couldn't make it. With little puffs of air and a pathetic voice, I heard myself saying, "I can't breathe." She told me to hang up and call the doctor to say I was coming in. The next thing I knew, she was at our doorstep ushering me into her car while Drew began walking down the alley to his brother's house. (I learned later that several times during the meeting, he wanted to leave, but they convinced him to stay.)

The cardiologist saw me right away, and when I told him about the gripping pain, he said he'd never heard of that happening from a cardioversion before. The EKG was fine, so the cardioversion had worked. He gave me two options: (1) to have a chest X-ray and bloodwork, or (2) go to the emergency room. I chose option one.

That evening, he called with the results and said the X-ray showed some signs of COPD. Well, that threw fear into me, because both of my parents were heavy smokers and died of COPD. I've never smoked even one cigarette but have had a morning "smoker's cough" for years. I guess second-hand smoke can be deadly too, but I'll think about that another day.

The achy pain and my inability to breathe lessened over the next week, and I was beginning to think I'd be fine for our grandson's wedding on October 17th. Daily, however, I could see and feel my weight climbing, and I was bloating up like a balloon. Nothing in my closet fit, not even the grandmother-of-the-groom dress I'd had altered the week before. Drew and I made it through the rehearsal and dinner on Friday night and enjoyed ourselves.

The wedding was held outdoors in chilly weather, and the ceremony was beautiful. Even though I got more short of breath with each step, I was able to guide Drew through all the paces of where to walk and when to sit. He got a little impatient having to wait for the photo session, and I was gasping for breath pretty much the whole time. But the doctor said my heart was in perfect sinus rhythm, so I figured it was just temporary. Drew wanted to leave the reception early, and I was pretty eager to get home myself.

In the wee hours, I couldn't breathe lying down, so I moved to the recliner next to the bed.

Was that a pinch I felt in my chest? Was that pressure in my chest? Should I call 911? No, I decided. It would be too confusing for Drew. It could wait until tomorrow, so I dozed off with the childhood bedtime prayer running through my mind: *If I should die before I wake, I pray the Lord my soul to take.*

October 18, 2015

Sunday morning, after Drew ate his breakfast and I had my wits about me, I had him drive me to the emergency room. He can still drive as long as he has someone to tell him where to turn.

I called Kim to meet us at the registration desk, and she saw Drew drop me off at the door and watched him park. The admission process was so efficient that the nurse had already ushered me into an examination room by the time Drew came in. Good thing Kim was there to sit with him and explain what the technicians were saying and doing. He had lots of questions, the most frequent being, "She'll be okay, right?"

The best answer she could give him was, "She's in the right place, and they're fixing her up."

I could see from his facial expression that her words were comforting to him. I knew they were comforting to me.

After discovering that the atrial flutter had returned, the ER doctor said they would give me some medicine that would have me back in rhythm in a couple of hours. Six hours later, when increasing doses of the magic medicine didn't touch my heart rate, he said, "It looks like we're going to have to give you another cardioversion."

"No way. I'm not having another one of those," I said. "It hurt me."

After the doctor had wiped the shock off his face, he arranged for my admission to the hospital.

We waited for hours for a bed to become available, and as evening approached, Drew became agitated and wanted to leave. One time, he just about marched out the door without so much as a wave goodbye. While Kim was trying to persuade him to stay, I said, "Hold on, buster, you're not getting out of here without giving me a kiss."

About that time Dana and Troy arrived, so they were able to calm him down. The next time he balked, Troy said he would drive him home.

"I can drive myself," Drew said.

It turned out that Kim went with them to the parking lot, and Drew allowed Troy to get behind the wheel without complaint. "You can just pull straight out," Drew told him. Troy put it in reverse. "No, Dad," he said. "If we pulled straight out, we'd wind up in that ditch."

(Note to self: Next time, call an ambulance.)

While our son-in-law, Wyatt, went to our house to get my CPAP machine, Kim kept me company in the ER while the clock continued to tick. We had a good visit with Wyatt when he dropped the bag off, and he said the grandkids were praying for me. Just hearing those words and being surrounded by my family gave me a fresh appreciation for how wonderful it is to be loved.

Kim told Wyatt to go on home because she wanted to stay with me until I got settled in my room, which didn't happen until 10:15. Knowing she had to be up early the next morning, I kept encouraging her to leave, but it pleased me that she insisted on being there.

After I had slept fitfully that night, the technicians ran a battery of tests on Monday. Dana brought Drew with her that morning, and Troy stopped by later in the day. Drew kept saying he needed to get home, but they persuaded him to wait and see what the doctors had to say. Knowing that they were monitoring him was a great comfort to me.

A team of cardiologists reviewed the results and agreed that another cardioversion wouldn't be effective for me. Instead, they recommended a cardiac ablation, a procedure that has a 99% success rate in resolving atrial flutter problems.

The nurse casually mentioned "congestive heart failure," and it took a while for me to realize she was talking about me. That sounded much more serious than a "flutter." I began to realize for the first time just how much trouble I was in.

On Tuesday, at 1:00 p.m., the nurses welcomed me back into the cardiac surgical unit where I'd had the cardioversion a few weeks earlier.

I stayed in the hospital overnight for observation, and on the morning of Wednesday, October 21st, I was discharged with a folder full of instructions—and one delighted husband.

Overall, Drew had been present throughout the whole ordeal, but he had no comprehension of the seriousness of it. He kept saying, "But you look fine. Everything's okay, isn't it?" And we all assured him that everything was going to be fine.

In the meantime, it has been a wake-up call for me to get some things in place if I'm suddenly out of commission. We've had our wills updated, but there are way too many loose ends like where the checkbooks are, who to notify, and a ton of other stuff. As soon as I'm strong enough, I'm going to have to make getting my "emergency plan" in place a top priority.

November 3, 2015

Drew is behaving as though I'm back up to speed, but I'm not there yet. I'm in the second week of wearing a heart monitor to track what feels like a fib (totally different than atrial flutter). The doctors assure me that we can treat it with medication, but it will just take some experimentation. My blood pressure has been way too low, vacillating between 77/52 and 82/44, making me dizzy whenever I stand up. If only I could be "me" again, with the energy to dig into all the things I've had to put aside. So far, I'm just concentrating on keeping the bills current.

Drew is very attentive, but last night he asked if we were somewhere else or were we home. I'm off balance in more ways than I can identify.

We got take-out from the Georgetown Family Restaurant. After dinner, Drew said, "I'll need to get you a key to the house." I assured him I had one, and he seemed satisfied. Later, while watching TV, he asked if I had any clothes or things I needed to get from somewhere else. I told him, "No, in fact, everything I own has been in this house for forty years."

He couldn't believe it and only became convinced when I showed him our wedding pictures.

Last week in the grocery store, he told me that if he were single, he'd have to come over and say something about how I caught his eye. I guess it started then. He's thrilled to discover that I belong to him and have for more than forty years.

November 5, 2015

Drew still can't comprehend that we're married; instead, he thinks we're dating. He woke me up the other morning at 5:50, shaking my shoulder, and saying with panic in his voice, "Candy, where am I supposed to meet you?"

Barely awake, I mumbled, "Right here in the bed where you belong."

"But what was I doing when you got here?"

"I don't know," I said. My sleep-filled mind hunted for an answer. "Working in the yard."

"No, I'm serious. What was I doing when you got here?"

"You were sleeping."

"Why didn't you wake me up when you got here?"

I didn't want to talk; I wanted to sleep. "Tired, I guess."

"I'm confused."

I buried my face in the pillow. "Me too. Let's get some sleep, and we'll figure it out in the morning."

Just as I was falling back to sleep, he said, "What time did you get here?"

"I've been here all along since we went to bed together last night. Let's go back to sleep."

"Okay. Good night."

"Good night, my love." I promised myself that I would pretend to be asleep if he said anything else, but sleep came quickly, and I didn't have to work at it.

CHAPTER EIGHT

Family Dinners
and Training Sessions

November 6, 2015

Tonight, he asked if I had met Troy.

Sadness swept over me. Troy was eleven when I "met" him. I told Drew I'd pretty much raised him, and he and Dana both look to me as a mother. He couldn't believe Troy's 51. Drew has misplaced the past forty years, but looking at the wedding album helped.

For the first time, he asked, "Is something wrong with my brain?" We had a long talk by candlelight about the brain tumor and the progressive damage it caused. He caught a glimmer of reality, and his first question was, "How are you doing with this? It has to have been hard on you."

"I'm doing fine. I've had a chance to get used to your short-term memory over the past several years, so it's been gradual for me. But this is a new stage, with you not being able to remember our forty years together. Just know this: If you ever want to know anything, just ask. That's what I'm here for—to fill in the blanks."

"And you're always going to be here?"

"Always. You're always here for me, and I'm always here for you. That's the promise we made when we said our vows forty years ago. You're mine, and I'm all yours, baby!"

Fifteen minutes later, when I said something about him not knowing we had been married for the past forty years, he didn't know what I was talking about. And so it goes. This is a good reminder for me to grab the lucid moments while I can.

We see the neurologist on December 14th, and I expect him to prescribe some additional medication for Drew.

November 7, 2015

People with dementia don't like change. Drew has never been much for change in the first place, but he's even more sensitive to it now. I replaced a night-light in the kitchen, and it now has a soft teal glow instead of yellow. As he settled into bed the first night, he asked where we were.

"Right here in our bed," I said.

"We're not on vacation in a hotel?"

Troy replaced our shower nozzle with one that has a water filter. What a wonderful difference it made for my skin and hair. For Drew, not so much. And the shower nozzle is much more personal than a night-light. The angle and the pressure of the spray of the old one was "just right," according to Drew. At first, I thought of asking Troy to put the old one back on but decided against it.

"This new nozzle has six settings," I said. "We'll keep experimenting and find one you like."

Although nothing else had changed in the shower, Drew suddenly didn't know which knob was hot and which one was cold. He didn't even know which side of the curtain to use, so I adjusted the water temperature for him and pulled back the curtain so he could get in.

Satisfied that he was able to bathe himself, I went to my office to catch up on a little work.

Twenty minutes later, all clean and dressed for bed, he came to get me. "I can't find it," he said. "Can you come help me?"

I didn't know what "it" was, and the best description he could give was, "You know, the thing. The thing in the shower."

It's not uncommon for us to play hide-and-seek. He hides, and I seek. It's a pretty predictable routine—usually his glasses or the remote control, but this one was a special challenge because I didn't know what I was looking for. He led me to the bathroom and pointed at the floor of the shower stall.

"Ahhh," I said as I gazed into the open hole. "The shower drain plug."

"Yeah. It was dirty, so I took it out."

And now, the metal drain catcher had disappeared. After searching in trash cans and every feasible place in the bathroom and bedroom, I was about to conclude that we were going to have to live temporarily with a gaping hole in the shower floor. But then he unwittingly gave me a clue.

"I would have taken it somewhere it would be easy to clean."

"Kitchen sink." I hurried to the one place I hadn't looked. There it was, all sparkly clean and snug, covering the garbage disposal hole.

November 9, 2015

Tonight Drew said, "Sometime, we should have a discussion about money."

Instead of jumping to conclusions, I said, "Wait a minute, let's light some candles and talk about it now in the kitchen." It turned out to be pretty much a repeat of the previous evenings, with a financial twist. He just couldn't comprehend that I've been coming through his front door for forty years when it seems to him like we only just met. That could be because we have so often replayed the day we met.

He said he was hesitant to ask me questions that might make me think less of him—that he wasn't "with it." I assured him that I respected him and then encouraged him to ask me anything, anytime, and we'd sit down together at the kitchen table and discuss it by candlelight.

"But what if I ask the same questions?" he said.

"Then I'll enjoy answering them all over again."

Candlelight discussions could become a very romantic routine.

November 10, 2015

I left a note: "Going to the drugstore and grocery store, so I'll be a while." For good measure, I added my cell phone number.

Who knew that a guide dog would have had a stinky accident in the pharmacy and that they would also be shorthanded, scrambling to find labels, only to discover that they were completely out? After I had stood for fifteen minutes in the stench-filled air, the guy in line ahead of me said he'd been waiting for more than an hour.

Who knew that I would sit in the car in the Walmart parking lot enjoying music on the radio for fifteen minutes in the rain—all the while trying to collect myself as I decided whether to go ahead and get the groceries? It took two hours to get everything on my list and then return to the drive-through window of the pharmacy for our medications even though I had pushed myself during the entire time.

When I pulled into the driveway, Buttercup was standing at the door wagging her tail, but Drew was sulking in the bedroom and didn't even come out like he's always done to help me bring in the bags.

He sat at the kitchen table and fired questions at me as I made trips to and from the trunk. "What took you so long?" "Where have you been?" "I was worried about you. Why didn't you call?"

My apology of "Sorry to have worried you" accelerated into an agitated back-and-forth that left me in tears. Finally, I sobbed, "I hear you. I got the message the first time, and you have told me ten times. I feel like you're scolding and punishing me. You can be sure of one thing: I will call you from now on, every fifteen minutes if you like." I could feel my heart pounding and didn't want it to escalate into twinges of pain, or worse. "I need to be calm for my heart," I shouted. Obviously, this was not the best way to get myself calm.

After I had cried myself out and finished putting the groceries away, exhaustion swept over me. Even so, I sat at the kitchen table with Drew and talked it out.

By bedtime, he was back to his favorite question: "How long have we been going together?"

"Forty years. We've been married forty years."

"And we've lived here in this house all those years?"

"Yep, right here in this house, loving and caring for each other."

It's a rare and precious thing to be courting again after all these years. Let the romance continue.

November 11, 2015

I had a stuffy nose and couldn't breathe through the CPAP machine I use for sleep apnea, so I settled into the recliner next to the bed—something I often do. For some reason, this time it agitated Drew because he wanted me lying next to him. I tried to explain, but nothing suited him except for me to move to my rightful spot in the bed. So I propped myself up with pillows the best I could, sitting pretty much straight up with my head unsupported. He insisted that I lie down like a normal person, which I tried but then felt suffocated and had to sit up again. So much for keeping calm.

He kept badgering me and finally I said, "Look, here's how it is. If I lie down, I can't breathe. And if I can't breathe, it puts stress on my heart, and you might wake up tomorrow and find me dead next to you, right here in the bed. Is that risk worth it to you?"

"What do you mean you have heart problems?" he said. "Why didn't you tell me?"

That calmed me down because I realized he didn't remember. I lowered my voice. "I thought you knew because you were the one who took me to the emergency room, and you were in the room and heard everything I did from the doctors and nurses."

For the rest of the night, he became the protector and defender of a husband I have always known. It wasn't long until he was fairly begging me to sleep in the recliner. "Look," he said, "this has a nice place to rest your head. You'll be much more comfortable here."

November 12, 2015

Last Friday, the doctor said if my blood pressure made me lightheaded again over the weekend, I should call 911 and get to the ER. I didn't have to do that, however, because it gradually crept up into the acceptable range. We still have to figure out how to get my irregular heartbeat to behave, but I have confidence the doctors will come up with a good solution, especially since an army of intercessors is praying for me.

Now and then, the words of a well-intended friend come to mind about the high percentage of caregivers who die before the ones they're caring for do. I don't want to be one of them.

Now that my blood pressure has come back into the normal range, I have lots of energy. I did some cleaning, ran a load of laundry, tried out my new pressure cooker, and invited Dana and John and Troy to dinner. The stimulation of conversation and interaction with others was really good for Drew. It just occurred to me how little exposure he has to other people these days.

My hope is to start a tradition of having small family groups here for dinner once a week so he can connect with everybody. Having six or less around the table is just right and not too confusing for him as with other family gatherings where there's a lot of commotion.

Kim and family are coming next week, and I'll invite the older grandchildren and their spouses, and then have another dinner with his brothers and their wives. Once a week should be just about right.

November 13, 2015

Dana and Troy came over for their first "training session" on what to do if something happens to me. We went over all of Drew's medications and their location, along with where I keep the checkbooks and the current bills. Then we covered a quick overview of a few other essentials. Drew sat quietly in a chair, listening as we went over everything and they took notes.

Before they left, we made an appointment to go to the banks and get their names on signature cards so they would be able to write checks. After that, we'll have a computer session about electronic banking, e-mailing my friends, and locating passwords for my online accounts.

Last year, after I got the wills, powers of attorney, and advance directives secured, I had these other things on my "should-do-this-soon" list. Since my brief hospital stay, however, "soon" has become "now." Indeed, sometimes we have to make time for the things we think we should do someday because someday it may be too late.

November 24, 2015

I couldn't sleep, so around 2:30 a.m., I propped myself up with pillows and turned on the light by my side of the bed. I'd been reading for about fifteen minutes when Drew stirred and got up to go to the bathroom. On his way back, he looked right at me and said, "Where's Candy?"

I waved my hands in the air and said, "Here I am!" and then motioned to the dog sleeping between us, "And here's Buttercup."

He looked puzzled as he slipped back into bed but didn't say anything. He just slipped under the covers and put his head on the pillow, facing me. For quite a while, I noticed he kept looking at me intently. *Oh, isn't that nice, he's thinking what a lucky man he is to have me.* Or maybe he's admiring me. I was wrapped up in my own little world of happy thoughts and high self-esteem.

But then he spoke. "Why are we sleeping together?"

Being certain that he was still having trouble remembering we've been married for forty years, I said, "Because that's what married people do."

And then he said, "But you're a man."

I didn't see *that* coming.

After recovering from the sting of his remark, I said, "Nope, I'm your wife. I'm all woman and have the female body parts to prove it," adding, "would you like to feel my boobies?"

Usually, that kind of playfulness would get a spark out of him, but he continued to half-frown and stare.

"You were dreaming. There was a man in your dream, and you think I'm the man. You're just not all the way awake yet."

"It was a dream?"

"Yes, just a dream."

He grunted, rolled over, and said, "Forget it," and was softly snoring a few seconds later.

I choose to think of this incident as sleepwalking, but it could be something more. It could be a foretaste of things to come when he looks at me and sees someone else. One of my prayers is that he will always know me. I continue to hope that the Lord will honor my request. My wise mother taught me years ago that God may not answer our prayers the way we want, but no matter what happens, He is always with us to give us strength and guidance when we need it. Surely, I'm experiencing the ultimate test of this truth.

December 6, 2015

Dana had a rough week. When she stopped by, we talked about how a lighthearted movie sometimes does the trick in resetting our perspective and clearing the emotional cobwebs out for us. Drew was with us last week when we looked online to see what movies would be playing on Sunday afternoon. We found a 3-D Disney movie, *The Good Dinosaur,* and he watched the trailer with us. When I asked if he would go with us, Drew said, "I'll go if John goes." I could see his mental wheels spinning. *John won't want to go, and Candy and I can stay home.* He is becoming more reclusive every day and feels happiest when it's just the two of us and our pets here at home, with no obligations to be anywhere or do anything.

But John agreed to go. For three days, I've been trying to condition Drew for our matinee outing—and for three days, he's grumbled about it.

Today is Sunday, and Drew says, "Why didn't you tell me? How can you expect me to do something like this on such short notice?" So we repeated the previous days' conversation for about the tenth time. "I don't want to go to a movie," he protested. "Why do I always have to do something I don't want to do?"

Okay, so it was time for me to be a little more firm. "You know, everything is not always about you and what *you* want. Sometimes we have to think about other people and what *they* want. Dana and John and I want to see this movie, and we'd like for you to go with us. Now, you can go to the movie with the three of us and then go out to dinner like a good boy, or you can stay home alone with Buttercup and miss out on the fun the rest of us are going to have."

It was risky. What if Drew had chosen to stay home? But it turns out I knew him as well as I thought I did. He would want to be with me wherever I was, and this time his manipulation hadn't convinced me to stay home. He said he'd go, and from then on the whining stopped.

December 9, 2015

Somebody said that if an author mentions a gun in a novel, then somebody has to get shot. But that's just a rule for fiction. This book is non-fiction, and nobody's going to get shot here. I bring up the subject of guns because Drew listens attentively to the news about ISIS and the homegrown terrorism threat and has been asking, "Where's the gun that Chief Todd gave me when he retired?"

"In the safe," I told him the first time he mentioned it. "But it's hard to get the combination to work, and it's late. We'll look into it tomorrow."

Drew is a protector by nature, and he had made up his mind that he needed to protect me. Day after day, he wanted to know where the gun was, and I repeated the same answer. On the fourth day, he said, "And don't tell me it's hard to get. Come with me right now and open the safe." It wasn't a request.

So much for my stall tactics. "Okay," I said, "but I'm not getting on my knees. You'll have to do that." Of course, he agreed, so I dutifully retrieved the combination and read the numbers to him s-l-o-w-l-y.

It took about five tries and some grumbling on his part, but the tumblers finally clicked into place, and the door opened when he twisted the handle. He held the .38 with satisfaction for a moment and then dug deeper into the safe. "Where are the bullets?"

Ahhh. I breathed a sigh of relief. "Sorry, hon, I guess we don't have any bullets. We'll have to look into that."

In the meantime, he decided that the gun should be closer to him at night in case anybody tried to "get us." He found a good hiding place in the bedroom.

He has asked about the bullets only one time since.

"We'll need to keep the bullets separate from the gun, you know," I said.

"Of course," he scowled. "Everybody knows that. It's basic gun safety."

I could see him start out that way and then think it would take too long to get the ammunition if he had to defend us. I can picture him deciding to move the bullets a little closer to the gun. And then it's a short mental step from there to deciding that it would take too long to load them into the chamber, and suddenly the empty gun would have live ammunition in it.

Drew has no concept of how slow his reaction time is or how much his muscle mass has weakened. In his mind, he still sees himself as the strong marksman who always hit the bull's-eye when target shooting, blowing cans off the fence with one blast after another.

A loaded gun in the hands of an Alzheimer's patient, no matter how well trained he once was, is a fearful thing. If bullets ever find their way into our bedroom, I'm going to have to make them disappear.

December 11, 2015

Our dear friend Doris saw us in a restaurant and sent a text message to me that evening: "Candy, I love the happiness I see in both of you."

I texted back, "Yes, we're more in love now than ever. I think it's a result of all those pats and kisses that have accumulated over the years."

It did my heart good to know that others see the joy that Drew and I have for each other. We laugh out loud when something strikes us funny, and we also play footsies under the table. Doris's comment made me realize something. When we first got married, we used to show affection for one another in private, but both of us have become more demonstrative in public over the last few years. It's almost as if Alzheimer's has given us permission to express our gratitude and be ourselves, enjoying one another wherever we are. And you know what? It makes the people around us happy, too.

December 14, 2015

I've been with Drew 24/7, but the tests they gave him at the neurologist's office revealed some surprises for me. When asked what year this is, he couldn't come up with an answer and said, "But I'll be able to write it down." On the paper, he wrote 19_ _ and then said, "That doesn't look right."

When asked, "Who's running for President?" he thought and thought and finally said, "The rich guy with the big mouth." The PA who administered the test and I exchanged looks and smiled because we knew he meant Donald Trump. When she asked, "What is his name?" he couldn't answer. His answer to her next question, "Who else is a candidate for President?" was "That's all. They can't get anybody else interested." *Hmmm.* He and I have been talking about Dr. Ben Carson for months, but he had no recollection of him or the personally autographed book he treasures.

She showed him a drawing of a seahorse, and he didn't know what it was, even when she gave him a hint that it lived in the ocean. When asked to identify a rhinoceros, he said it looked like some sort of bulldog. And when she said, "Do you know what this is?" and showed him a drawing of a unicorn, he said, "That's a horse." She pointed at its long horn. "And what's this?" He frowned and said, "I don't know, but I'll tell you this—no horse of mine would ever have one of those!"

During the last visit, when he was asked to write a sentence, he wrote, "I love my wife." This time he wrote, "This is not fun," and whispered to me, "She's trying to trick me."

I sensed that Drew would freak out if someone confronted him about the diagnosis, so I requested in advance of the appointment that the neurologist not mention Alzheimer's to him. He did an excellent job of referring to the meningioma (benign brain tumor) removed from his frontal lobe a few years ago as the culprit for his memory lapses.

The doctor talked about the importance of physical exercise and instructed me to be firm about engaging Drew in mental activities like puzzles, cards, and other games that would stretch his mind beyond his comfort zone. Since Drew used to be a Pontiac dealer, he asked him about different models of Pontiacs, but he couldn't come up with any. So one mental exercise we might try is flash cards with pictures of the cars he used to sell.

The doctor mentioned a new medication in the final stages of testing by Lilly Pharmaceuticals that looks very promising. If all goes well, it should be available in the next year or two. Fingers crossed.

When we left the office, I told Drew that he did an excellent job with all those hard questions and the doctor didn't prescribe any more pills.

"So, it was a good visit?" he asked.

"Yes," I said, as the automatic door opened. Hand in hand, we walked out of the building into balmy 73° December weather and played golden oldies on the radio all the way home.

Watch your thoughts,
for they may break out into words
at a moment's notice.

—Anonymous

CHAPTER NINE
A Summary Sheet

December 22, 2015

Yesterday, Drew asked me, "What is your full name?"

"Candace Louise Fennemore Abbott," I said. "Why do you ask?"

"It's important that I know these things. When's your birthday?"

I smiled. "June 7th. Any other questions?"

"How old are you?"

"Sixty-eight. Last week you asked me to make a copy of my driver's license, and I put it on your dresser so that you can look at it anytime you want. But feel free to ask me anything at any time. I'm your full-service answer lady."

"How old am I?"

"You'll be eighty in March."

This morning he asked me where I live. When I told him this is my home and that we've been married for more than forty years, he was once again surprised and delighted.

The strange thing about all this is that I'm no longer caught off guard when he doesn't know basic things. It used to be like a knife to my heart, so I guess I'm adapting to our new reality. When he sees other people, he asks them how they're doing and lets them do the talking. Afterward, they tell me that he seems "just fine."

He got concerned about what he would give me for Christmas. I told him that I only wanted two things—a self-sharpening knife set and pajamas—and assured him I had ordered them online for him so he wouldn't have to mess with traffic and shoppers.

I got out the wrapping paper and asked if he would wrap them for me. He liked that. But it didn't take long before he asked me for help. Side by side, we wrapped my presents. He held the paper steady while I taped the package, and voila! Candy's Christmas presents were ready to place under the tree.

Five minutes later, he asked, "What do you want for Christmas? I have to get you something."

I showed him the newly wrapped packages, and then he said, "That's fine, but I think I'll give you money so you can get whatever you want." So I wrote out a check for him to cash when I drive him to the bank. At least he can still walk into the bank and up to the teller without my assistance, but I'm still keeping a close eye on him.

December 23, 2015

Just like Drew keeps asking (now more than once a day) how long we've been "going together," he has a new favorite question: "Can you get pregnant?" It's not every day that a sixty-eight-year-old woman gets to educate a seventy-nine-year-old man on the phenomena of menopause. Or perhaps it will be like this every day since this is a question I've heard more than once already.

He seemed surprised that I dressed in my pajamas instead of putting on my coat and said, "You're staying overnight?"

"Yes, indeed," I said as I reached for the calculator. "Let's see . . . according to my calculations, I've been sleeping with you now for 14,782 nights."

He liked that and asked me to write it down so he could look at it. Even so, he still can't comprehend that we're married and have been for forty-plus years.

December 31, 2015

With the flurry of this year's Christmas activities behind us, I'm approaching the New Year with the need to take better care of myself. Several incidents have opened my eyes to the fact that the pattern of catering to Drew's wishes day in and day out in an attempt to keep him happy would result in the loss of my identity if I'm not careful.

On Christmas Eve, I waited until it was time to get dressed to tell him. "We're going to the candlelight service at church, and by the way, Howard and Kelly will be having their annual party afterward."

As I expected, he responded, "Why can't I just stay home and do what I want to do?"

"Because it's Christmas and it's important for the family to be together."

More grumbling.

"Okay," I said. "Here's the deal. Trevor and Jill and Troy and I are going to church, and then we're going to Howard and Kelly's. You can stay here by yourself, or you can get dressed and go with us. Either way, I'm going."

He blinked and, by George, he got it. "If you're going, I'm going with you."

It's been months since we've been in church, and I think it felt good for him to sit in the pew. Other than turning to leave by way of the choir room instead of the lobby area, he did fine.

We went to the party. Drew was pleasant to the thirty-some people who milled around, but he didn't recognize most of them. At one point, he asked about the handsome guy in the green shirt. "Is he married to somebody important?"

"He sure is," I said. "That's Wyatt, our son-in-law. He's married to my daughter, Kim, and she's important to us."

A minute later, as more family members came into the room, he said, "Howard and Kelly sure do have a lot of friends."

On Christmas Day, our immediate family of eleven others came for brunch, and Drew wasn't as bothered by the commotion as I had anticipated. He did one subtle thing that expressed his dependency on me: Instead of taking his usual seat at the opposite end of the dining room table, he asked where I would be sitting and sat next to me. It was kind of nice to sit side by side where I could pat his knee beneath the tablecloth.

The Fennemores (my side of the family) reserve December 27th for our Christmas reunion in Camden, Delaware. As I was preparing my chicken/broccoli casserole, Drew fussed about having to go somewhere again and wanted to know why people always had to eat when they got together. Hmmm . . . I wasn't sure how to answer that except to say, "That's what people do."

Drew seemed in good spirits as we drove from home to Bart and Clea's house, and when we got there, he found a quiet spot on the couch and settled in. The hubbub in the great room increased while more and more of the family arrived with food, hugs, and piles of gifts. He seemed relaxed even in the midst of the rising levels of conversation and squeals of delight as the little ones raced around. We ate in the dining room, and as soon as he was finished eating, he said, "We can go now, right?"

I was able to stall for a while. Late afternoon turned to early evening, and I could tell from the set of his jaw that Drew was getting tense and wanted to leave. After dismissing my fearful thoughts of him "sundowning," I told him, "Not yet. The kids haven't opened their presents, and we're going to have a group picture and sing carols."

When we moved back into the living room and the children were in full swing unwrapping gifts, he said, "This is for kids. We don't have to be here, do we?"

"Just a little longer, hon," I said. "I want to see them open our gifts."

They had barely finished when Drew began fidgeting and becoming agitated. I took one look at his face and saw something that resembled panic, so I said, "We can go now." As I offered hasty, apologetic goodbyes, Kade and Saige helped take our stuff to the car. The next thing I knew, Drew and I were out the door and had taken two steps down the brick walkway when he said, "I have to go to the bathroom," so back inside we went.

I had steeled myself to the need to leave. But surrounded once more by the loving presence of my brothers and their families, tears welled up. I couldn't hold them back. Suddenly, I had a "want." I wanted to be with my family. I wanted to enjoy their company, to sing with them, to linger over stories, and to laugh. Instead, I knew that we needed to leave.

Bart said, "You look like you could use a prayer. Would you like me to pray for you?"

"Oh, yes," I whimpered.

He wrapped his arm around my shoulder and whispered the most comforting, reassuring prayer in my ear. I felt the Lord's presence, and by the time he finished praying, my soul was at peace.

I drove the long way home, around Andrew's Lake, to see the house where Mom and Dad had lived, trying to milk another moment of nostalgia from the evening. They both died a long time ago, and the house looks all different now with other people living there, but it did give me one more morsel of family closeness. It was a bittersweet reminder that life is fleeting and we only have "this moment."

One thing Alzheimer's does is force us to live in the moment. The key, I decided, is to make the most of the moments we have, entering into them with all their realities—the tender ones as well as those that grate on our nerves.

That night, as I was savoring the day, Drew said, "I knew there was something I wanted to mention. What was that about with that guy hugging and kissing on you?"

"What guy?"

"Don't deny it," he said. "When I came out of the bathroom, I know what I saw. Some guy had his arm around you, and he was kissing you."

"That was Bart, my *nephew*, and he was *praying* for me."

"It doesn't matter who he is. He was kissing you!" he insisted. "How far does this go?"

"You can stop right there." Fury exploded within me for the unjust accusation, but I managed to keep calm. The scene with

Bart—as comforting, pure, and holy as it was to me—obviously touched a jealous nerve in Drew, who couldn't separate his perception from the reality of what happened. "You're trying to make something beautiful into something ugly, and I will not let you ruin it."

"You think there was nothing wrong with what he did?"

"That's right." I forced myself to sound lighthearted. "Bart did nothing wrong and everything right, and no amount of badgering will get me to say any different."

"So you would let him do it again?"

"Yes, I would do it again. I would be delighted to have Bart pray for me again."

"Don't lie to me. He was hugging and kissing you. I know what I saw." Drew was in output mode and unable to hear or comprehend anything I said.

And so it went for hours. Eventually, I convinced him that my affection was reserved totally and completely for him alone. We went to sleep holding hands with a silent prayer on my lips for Drew to forget this whole distorted incident.

January 1, 2016

Our teenage grandchildren haven't spent the night at our house in a long time, and Christmas vacation seemed like a good time to try. Kade, my almost six-foot, fifteen-year-old grandson, is very affectionate, so I had to caution him not to scratch my back whenever Drew is around so he won't accuse "that man" of touching me. So sad, but he understands.

January 4, 2016

Lately, whenever we're shopping at Walmart, Drew follows behind me as I push the cart, so I have to keep looking over my shoulder to make sure he's still with me. As we rounded the corner, I glanced back, and he said, "Want to have some fun? The next Walmart worker you see, tell him, 'I don't know who this guy is, but he keeps following me.'"

We were still laughing when I noticed the husband of one of my publishing clients in the same aisle. We greeted one another, and I asked Drew if he remembered Keith. He said no, and they both shook hands. Keith began chatting with me about his wife's books and his new teaching job, and I could feel Drew getting fidgety standing beside me.

After a few minutes, Drew walked away, so I said a quick goodbye to Keith and caught up with him by the frozen foods. His body language told me that he was not happy.

"How long could you stand there talking to that guy?" he wanted to know. Before I could answer, he said, "He never said a word to me or looked at me the whole time. Who is he, anyway?"

"That's Keith, remember? And he did speak to you when you shook hands."

"I didn't shake anybody's hand," he said with a grunt.

I stopped pushing the cart and looked at him. "You did, hon, a few minutes ago when I introduced you. Your memory must be short-circuiting again." I looked at my list and said, "The last thing on my list is bacon—it's right over there." End of discussion, thank You, Lord.

The lesson I learned from this scene is that Drew doesn't like to be ignored. I can't blame him. Who does?

January 5, 2016

Dr. Edelsohn had given me strict instructions to do things with Drew that would challenge him mentally. When Kade and Saige spent the night, Dana stopped in, and the four of us convinced him to join us for bingo. He played a couple of cards and then got bored, so he watched TV while we started another game. Then we played Phase Ten and Uno into the night.

As I was getting ready to put the pack of playing cards away today, I remembered Dr. Edelsohn's admonition that it was up to me to find ways to stimulate his brain.

"How about a quick game of cards?" I asked.

For someone who was never interested in any games except checkers, he surprised me when he said, "Sure, but you'll have to teach me."

We played four hands of Uno, and both of us won two games. It surprised me to find out that he didn't know the suits. Even when I coached him on clubs, spades, diamonds, and hearts, he got them confused. Like a child, he would show me his card and ask if it matched. It was slow going, but at least he was willing.

January 6, 2016

Drew is struggling to realize that we're married and have been for more than four decades. The marker board I used on December 23rd was getting smeared, so I typed up this page for him last night that addresses most of the questions he asks:

We've been sleeping together for 14,580+ nights and enjoying each other the same number of days (forty and a half years).

Your Aunt Fannie, who was my daughter's babysitter at the time, walked me across the street from her house to yours and introduced us on a balmy evening in May 1975. You proposed to me three weeks later on my twenty-eighth birthday (June 7th). At the time, Dana was fifteen, Troy was eleven, and Kim was three and a half. We began renovating the house immediately. Rev. Jim Mays married us in the Georgetown Presbyterian Church on Saturday, June 29, 1975. In September, we held a big reception in our backyard.

Today, we're "living happily ever after," as all good fairy tales go.

He read the paper aloud three times and then put it on the desk in the bedroom. We had a long talk about his memory loss, and I could tell from the concern he expressed that he's beginning to grasp the reality of his situation.

"It seems like you're being cheated," he said. "You deserve better than this."

"That's funny," I said. "I've always felt like you were too good to be true and I didn't deserve you. I still feel that way. You're the best thing that's ever happened to me, and I'll take you any way I can get you."

The tension on his face melted away.

"Whether you can remember anything or not, you're still you—your kind, generous, protective, compassionate self. The most important thing," I said, looking deep into his eyes, "is that you love me, and I love you. And no matter what happens, I'm here, and I'm not going anywhere. This is my home, and you are my life."

This morning, the first thing Drew said was, "What's going on? Did we get married? I have a ring on my finger."

"That's right—we got married. Let me get something that should answer all your questions." I located the paper, and he read it at the kitchen table while I fried eggs and put the bread in the toaster.

"I must have asked this before," he said when he put the paper down.

"Yes, last night we had a long talk about your memory, and I typed that up for you."

He took a sip of coffee. "But what happens if I ask again and again?"

"Every time you ask, I'll get the paper, and you can have a refresher course. It's like we're in a perpetual courtship where everything is new again."

With that, his sense of humor showed up. He broke into song, hitting every note of "Getting to Know You" perfectly. How I wish I had caught it on videotape so I could watch his exaggerated facial expressions and look of sincerity! Oh, to replay it over and over.

January 7, 2016

Doris has been helping me clean, but the house needs extra support to get into all the nooks and crannies we don't have time or energy to tackle. So I lined up a highly recommended cleaning service to come in, and Brandon of B Dun Cleaning came this morning.

Drew came out to meet him and then retreated to the bedroom where he sulked and fussed with me because "he's a man." He tried to get me to say that it would be a one-time thing, but I stood my ground because I'll need Brandon's services on a monthly basis.

I stayed with Drew in the bedroom, watching TV and listening to him badger me for the next two hours. When I got tired of giving him the same answers, I closed my eyes and then dozed off. When I woke up, he was cheerful and even thanked Brandon for his good work when he left.

I told him we should celebrate having a clean house by going to Red Lobster, where we had a lovely dinner and lighthearted conversation. Then we visited PetSmart to get dog food.

When we got home, I was just about to put the key in the lock when I heard a crash behind me. Drew, carrying a bag of food in each hand, had fallen into the bushes. His shoe must have missed the first step, and down he went. He rolled into the fall instead of resisting (which may have been an instinctive muscle memory reaction from his high school football days) and only wound up with a small cut on his cheek.

He showered and seemed to be handling it well, so we took out the trash together—one bag for me and one for him. (Our new rule: he's only allowed to carry one thing at a time from now on.) Buttercup was on her lead by the back door, and as we rounded the corner by the millstone, she ran in front of him, stretching the lead taut, and Drew almost tripped over it. If he had fallen that time, he would have landed face down. We'd better get that millstone lamp fixed pronto because that corner of the yard is dark. I guess we're child-proofing the house all over again—for big people.

I'm going to have to keep a closer eye on him.

January 9, 2016

Drew delights in setting up "gotcha" moments but hasn't been able to trip me up lately. Tonight, he stood beside me at the kitchen counter as I fixed a snack of cheddar and Triscuits. I sliced the cheese and put it on a paper towel with a handful of crackers for us to share. When I put the leftover cheese back in the refrigerator, Drew took all the Triscuits but one and hid them behind his back, and then he waited to see my reaction. I stopped short and gasped when I saw the empty paper towel, and he howled with laughter. So did I—not only from the joke he'd played on me but from sheer joy that his playfulness and humor are still intact, something I have loved about him from the start.

*You can't speak a kind word too soon
for you never know how soon it will be too late.*

—Ralph Waldo Emerson

CHAPTER TEN

Care for the Caregiver

January 11, 2016

I'm reading *Caregiving Our Loved Ones: Stories and Strategies That Will Change Your Life* by Nanette J. Davis, Ph.D., which I highly recommend. It's an easy read, and every page is insightful. In chapter 9, she quotes Sandy Stork, a mental health specialist working with families dealing with Alzheimer's.

> The caregiver's dilemma is this: She cannot leave her beloved charge, while, at the same time, the physical and emotional demands are too often excessive. This sets the stage for unremitting stress. Non-stop stress is not a benign condition.
>
> From a scientific perspective, the chronic stress response is dangerous. The overproduction of cortisol directly impacts the adrenal glands—the system that regulates our stress hormones—and the result is constant fatigue, emotional exhaustion, and lowered immune response. In fact, chronic stress plays some part in all illnesses. An

Ohio State University study found that older caregivers of family members with dementia did not respond well to vaccines, had fewer defenses against viruses as well as more inflammation and accelerated aging of their cells compared with adults who were not caregivers.

Sandy Stork recommends that caregivers view themselves as CEOs, chief executive officers, in their management of self and their care receiver. The process starts with a strong identity, a positive self-image, and a set of practices that enhance well-being. Sandy recommends three basic—not always easy—stress reduction practices:

1. *Change your approach to the care receiver*—show a happy face.
2. *Alter your routines to include taking care of yourself.* Certainly, you are as important as the loved one. Keep a schedule book to include regular activities that can renew and refresh you. Where have you been on your calendar?
3. *Reach out to others, including friends, family and support groups.* Talk to someone you love or admire every day to re-energize yourself.

She goes on to say that grief has a life of its own, which needs to be embraced and never repressed. "Your task is to recognize these feelings and work with them, *listening* to them and *responding appropriately.*"

In light of these things, on a scale from 1 to 10, I'd give myself an overall score of 8 (happy face) and a 2 for taking care of myself (diet, exercise, and stress management). I've signed up for a ten-week Beth Moore Bible study that starts this Wednesday. Hopefully, that will reconnect me face-to-face with praying friends, give me solid spiritual food, and get me out of the house at least once a week.

January 14, 2016

Attending yesterday's Bible study was like "coming home" to sit around the table with seven other believers. The topic is "The Fruit of the Spirit," based on Galatians 5:22-23 (which is my life Scripture). Since this particular study has a workbook, I'll be "plugged in" during the week.

My next endeavor to do something for myself involves attending a writing retreat this weekend. For more than a decade, I've joined with eleven people from seven states (Delaware, Illinois, Maryland, New Jersey, New York, Pennsylvania, and Tennessee), informally known as "The Crue," who serve as mentors to one another for our writing and our lives. Over this long period, we've thoroughly bonded with one another.

I've been preparing all week by charging my laptop, printing papers, gathering things to pack—but mostly trying to get Drew conditioned to the idea so he can handle my being away for two days and one night.

The weekend is usually three days and two nights, but I'm only staying one night this year because Drew panicked last year and called me four times in the wee hours of the second night not knowing where I was and upset that I wasn't in his bed. When I got home, I found the note I had carefully prepared with all the essential details buried beneath a pile of mail. No wonder he didn't know what I meant when I told him to look at the note on the bar in the kitchen.

This time I've made several copies of the note and already posted them on the microwave, his bathroom mirror, and the back door:

Friday, January 15th

I'm leaving around 2:00 to be with Nancy Rue and my writing mentors on the other side of the Bay Bridge, near Annapolis. I'll be spending the night. Feel free to call me at any time (my cell phone).

Saturday, January 16th

We have workshops that go through Saturday afternoon. My plan is to leave around 5:00 and be home by 7:00, but that might change. I'll call to let you know how things are going, and you can always call me (my cell phone).

I've also written detailed notes about how to feed the cat and the dog (because he gets their food mixed up) and have coached him to do it himself. He still doesn't know for sure which container has the dog food, even though I put the canned cat food on the counter with a note saying, "This is for the cat." When I'm not looking, he puts the dry *dog* food in the kitty's bowl, and I expect Buttercup will feast on canned cat food while I'm gone.

I put Drew's medications in baggies labeled "Friday 9 PM" and "Saturday 10 AM" and gave them to Troy so he can make sure Drew takes them when he should. Drew pooh-poohed the idea and said he could take his own medicine, so I told him, "Let's give the job to Troy because it'll make him feel important." I later shared this with Troy, and we both had a good chuckle.

Dana and Troy will have dinner with Drew on Friday and Saturday, and Kim will check on him, too. I'll call Drew often. I'm hoping for a relaxing, inspirational couple of days for myself and an enjoyable time for Drew and the kids.

January 15, 2016

I received an e-mail from Breakthrough, an intercessory prayer organization, with the following prayer from the archives of Catherine Marshall. Although Catherine never knew it, she served as my writing mentor because her books inspired me to keep a prayer journal that served as a springboard for my first book. With my weekend writing retreat before me, this is her timely reminder that God is in control of His plans and purposes.

"Give Me a Dream"

Father, once—it seems long ago now—I had such big dreams, so much anticipation of the future. Now no shimmering horizon beckons me; my days are lackluster. I see so little of lasting value in the daily round. Where is Your plan for my life, Father?

You have told us that without vision, we men perish. So Father in heaven, knowing that I can ask in confidence for what is Your expressed will to give me, I ask You to deposit in my mind and heart the particular dreams, the special vision You have for my life.

And along with the dream, will You give me whatever graces, patience, and stamina it takes to see the dream through to fruition? I sense that this may involve adventures I have not bargained for. But I want to trust You enough to follow even if You lead along new paths. I admit to liking some of my ruts. But I know that habit patterns that seem like cozy nests from inside, from Your vantage point may be prison cells. Lord, if You have to break down any prisons of mine before I can see the stars and catch the vision, then Lord, begin the process now.

In joyous expectation, Amen.

At 2:00, I loaded my suitcase, laptop bag, and groceries into the trunk, and went back into the house to tell Drew I was ready to leave. Instead of wrapping his arms around me and praying as he usually does, he had retreated to the bedroom. I found him sitting in his recliner.

"I'm leaving now." I expected him to get up and at least kiss me goodbye.

Instead, he just sat there and said, "Have a good time."

I motioned for him to get up, which he did.

"You're not going to let me out of this house without a kiss, are you?"

Then he gave me a perfunctory kiss. Instead of walking me to the car and waving until I was out of sight, he sat down and said, "Watch the crazy drivers."

I felt a sense of sad freedom as I drove without incident to Brenda Ulman's, where she and Pam Halter came running out to greet me and help carry my bags inside. Remembering the many enjoyable and inspiring annual meetings of "The Crue" at Brenda's, I felt the stress begin to melt away the moment I nestled myself on the couch.

That night at dinner, with Nancy Rue and the others around the table, I shared the John Smith's Bay story about Drew and his underpants, and we all had a good laugh. When I told them that I was capturing scenes that would someday be part of a book entitled, *I've Never Loved Him More*, they offered resounding affirmation.

Someone said, "This has to be hard for you."

Often I write with tears flowing, but now, unexpected words bubbled out of me. "It's not hard at all."

There was a collective gasp around the table. "Huh? What do you mean it's not hard?"

I rushed to explain. "I have a rare opportunity to love my husband as I've never loved him before—to appreciate him and each day we have together. It's an honor and a blessing to do for Drew what he can't do for himself."

And then I backpedaled a bit. "Well, it was hard at first, and I'm sure I'll have hard days ahead, but I'm learning to rely more on God's grace than on myself." The phrase in Psalm 34:14, "Seek peace and pursue it," has always meant a lot to me. By pursuing peace for *him*, I'm finding peace for *me*, the kind of peace I could never manufacture on my own—the kind of peace that passes human understanding.

January 16, 2016

When I called Drew in the morning, he told me about having an oyster stew with Dana and Troy the night before and asked if I had lined up any plans for him that day.

"None in particular," I replied.

"Well, if anybody shows up, I'll just do what they say," he said and seemed happy about that.

Our theme for the retreat was "Enthusiasm," and each of the workshops contained Scriptures and exercises providing opportunities for soul searching and sharing.

"And at this stage, I can say that I'm enthusiastic about being able to focus on Drew. I don't know how long we'll have together, but I cherish him every day, whether he knows it or not. I like to think that the tone I'm setting is helping to keep his tenderhearted temperament intact.

"Adding little snippets to the manuscript is cathartic for me. I've also learned to send up quick little 'help' prayers, and the Lord never fails to hand down an extra measure of contentment.

"The Alzheimer's challenge became a lot easier when I stopped trying to work harder at it (whatever 'it' was at any given moment). But this didn't come easy," I said.

Then I shared how a visit from my friend Barry Jones gave my mindset a paradigm shift:

While I was recovering from my heart issues, Barry stopped by to give me a copy of her son DaRain Powell's book, *Heavy Call, Lonely Walk*. The moment she hugged me, I began to cry and pour out my woes.

"I miss my Christian sisters," I said. "Your visit is like manna from heaven." She enveloped me in her arms, and my complaints came pouring out: "I don't have lunch with friends, attend prayer groups or conferences, go to Bible study, or lead Mothers With a Mission anymore, and I'm pulling away from Delmarva Christian Writers' Fellowship. Drew needs me with him because I'm his lifeline, and I've given up everything that takes my time and attention away from him."

The more I rambled, the more the tears flowed. "I feel unplugged from the body of Christ," I sobbed. "It's like I'm all alone—like I'm in some sort of wilderness, and I can't find my way out."

"Honey," Barry said as we sat down. "Read the back cover."

"What?"

"The book in your hand. Read the back cover of DaRain's book."

It took a moment for my vision to focus due to the tears, and I gasped as I read the first four words of the first line:

> Moses in the wilderness, David in the valley, Daniel in the lion's den. When you have a heavy call on your life, God will bring you to a lonely place so He can deal with everything about you—body, soul, and spirit. Jesus was alone a lot.

Barry's eyes were soft. "Candy, the greater the call on your life, the greater the wilderness experience."

I cried harder. But these tears came from the freedom, joy, and hope I felt as I realized that my wilderness experience was meant for a good purpose, not a punishment or exile. This wilderness is *intentional.* Instantly, my perspective changed, and praise bubbled up within me filling the empty places that had been there just moments before.

God is faithful. I can count on Him to complete the good work He began in me with my writing, my publishing, the ministries I had founded, and my faith journey.

"From that moment on," I told the Crue, "I saw Drew through new eyes. I realized that I have him all to myself—I get to love him as he deserves to be loved without being preoccupied. What a rare privilege to have this opportunity to appreciate and serve him in a deeper way than *ever* before."

The Crue celebrated Communion that afternoon, and I felt lighter and filled with a deeper kind of peace than when I arrived at Brenda's on Friday.

I left at 4:00 and had a quick and delightfully uneventful drive home.

Drew was even-keeled and eagerly waiting to go to dinner, so I was able to enjoy the weekend with no repercussions. I now feel refreshed.

The kids said they enjoyed spending time with their dad. Since this worked so well, maybe I can plan a private overnight respite next month to regain the time for solitude I used to take for granted.

January 17, 2016

Drew's brother Tim is having a "70th Birthday Open House" today. When the time came to get ready, Drew said, "What? Birthday parties are for kids."

I smiled and said, "No, birthday parties are for anybody who is not dead. Now, go get dressed."

And so began the litany of reasons he should stay home:

"It's snowing."

"It's just a dusting," I said.

"The roads are dangerous."

"I'll be extra careful driving," I said.

"People will want to talk."

"Just be polite and nod," I said.

And on and on we went, back and forth, while the clock kept ticking. Finally, I'd had enough. "Myrna has prepared some wonderful food. It's open house, so we don't have to stay the entire time. You can just say happy birthday to Tim, have a nice lunch, and then we can leave. But you need to be there."

He gave me a lopsided smile. "Okay. How about if I just sit in the car?"

I pictured him in the car peeping out the window, and suddenly the whole conversation seemed hilarious. Did you know that a good belly laugh will change the atmosphere in a room?

At the party, he wanted me to sit beside him on the couch, which I did while we ate. Then I stood up and chatted with people in the same room. His friend, Carlton Moore, took my seat and talked with Drew for some time. I'd glance over periodically, expecting Drew to give me an "it's-time-to-leave" signal, but I found him fully engaged in conversation with Carlton. He didn't even notice me.

Sometimes, just being in the company of others can breathe life into a person. I know our brief time at the party did that for me.

January 18, 2016

As we shared cups of hot chocolate this morning in the kitchen, Drew noticed that the sky was particularly blue. "Why is the sky blue?" he asked.

"I don't know. When we get to heaven, we'll have to ask God about that."

He sipped his cocoa and then, without a word, pushed his chair back from the table and stood in front of the sliding glass doors. He was quiet for a long time while staring at the sky, and I didn't say a word.

And then he spoke. "I just asked God why the sky is blue. Do you want to know what He said?"

"Yes, of course."

"He said, 'Can you think of a better color?'"

We agreed that God is the Great Designer and must have had fun figuring out all the details when He created our world and everything around us.

January 20, 2016

Last night Drew asked me to write my name so he could have it for reference if anything happened.

"Do you want me to sign it or print it?"

"Maybe you should do both," he said.

We went to bed around 10:00, and at midnight, I coughed and stirred.

"Are you awake?" Drew asked.

"Not really. Why?"

"Who are you?"

The question I've been dreading jolted me awake.

"I'm Candy. I'm your wife."

Apparently, instead of sleeping, he had been trying to figure this out for two hours. So *that's* why he wanted me to write my name.

I got up and searched for our marriage certificate to prove we're husband and wife because he thought I was making it up.

We went through our been-married-forty-years dialogue and discussed the benign brain tumor that caused his memory loss. Then I said, "You'll know me in the morning. Your memory problems are worse at night."

And this morning, he did know me again. He's in the kitchen whistling, humming, and—of all things—yodeling.

Please, Lord, keep him happy and let him always know me.

Life is what we make it.
Always has been, always will be.

— Grandma Moses

CHAPTER ELEVEN

Learning To See Through His Eyes

January 21, 2016

We have an appointment tomorrow morning with Procino-Wells & Woodland, elder law specialists, to make sure we're doing all we can to prepare for whatever comes. A few weeks back, I filled out a questionnaire that Drew signed, and he was on board with this appointment at the time. But tonight, when I set the alarm clock and he asked why, he dredged up the whole situation about the will that we resolved a year and a half ago (which, of course, he couldn't remember).

I gave the simplest explanation I could. "This isn't about the will. This is a meeting with an attorney who specializes in old people—you are about to turn eighty—and we want to know all the options available to make sure we're protecting our assets."

Instantly, Drew returned the conversation to the will and his dormant concerns, so I had to think fast to keep him out of distress mode.

"Tomorrow is not about the will. We got that squared away in 2014 when you and Dana and Troy and I sat around this table and thrashed out all the details. When we got done, you were completely satisfied. You're happy about the will. You just don't know it."

About that time, Drew glanced out the sliding glass door and saw Buttercup with her lead caught on the corner of the deck. It's January. It's cold. It's windy. But instead of getting up as usual, he just sat there and said, "She's hung up."

Eager for an escape from our conversation, I jumped up. "I'll get her. You have more important things to worry about."

He laughed, and the rest of the night was peaceful.

Fortunately, Dana will go with us tomorrow, so I won't be alone as we tread into unknown territory with the attorney about elder law matters.

January 22, 2016

When I woke Drew up at 7:00, told him he had an hour to get ready, and explained where we were going, he decided he'd rather roll over, go back to sleep, and stay home. "You and Dana understand this stuff better than I do," he said. "Why don't you two go and tell me later what you find out."

I'm so glad it worked out this way because the conversation was complex, detailed, and difficult for *us* to comprehend. Drew would have asked so many questions and wouldn't have been able to understand the answers. Stress would have consumed me.

As it turned out, Dana and I quickly realized that the fees are well worth the services their firm has to offer, so we'll be making the investment and following up. Our next appointment is in February, and I want all three kids to go with me so they can hear firsthand everything that I learn. As the saying goes, "Two heads are better than one"—or in this case, four heads are better than two. I'm so grateful that we are in one accord and can trust one another. Not all families are so fortunate.

February 5, 2016

Over the past few days, I've noticed a few little things I want to share.

When Drew and I got married, we converted the den into the master bedroom and remodeled the back porch to be our bathroom. Drew has difficulty coming up with the right names for certain items, so he'll say, "You know, that *thing*." But when he referred to our bedroom as the den, I realized that not only did he not know the right name for the bedroom but mentally he was still stuck in the '70s after his divorce and before our marriage.

That explains why he thinks we're dating and asks, "Have you stayed overnight before?" It also clarifies why he asks again which side of the bed he sleeps on and says things like, "When you've been living alone as long as I have, it's hard to change."

He's good-natured and compliant, so that's a blessing I'm hoping will continue. It's like we're in a perpetual courtship in which every kiss is like a *first kiss*. We're truly living in the moment—which, of course, is the best way to live in the first place.

The day before yesterday, he stood in the doorway of my home office with a belt in his hand and announced that he was going to take Buttercup for a walk.

"Oh," I said, as my mind raced to find the right words. "Then you're going to need her leash."

He looked perplexed at the belt in his hand as if it had somehow played a magic trick on him, while our cocker spaniel danced around in anticipation at his feet.

"Come on," I smiled, "I know right where it is." So he followed me like a puppy to the place where we keep the leash.

Yesterday, as we were eating lunch in a restaurant. People were sitting in the booth behind him, and a man with his back to us was at another table. Drew made a couple of playful remarks in a louder-than-he-realized voice.

I scowled. "You have to stop saying inappropriate things in public. People can hear you."

He looked remorseful. "What things?"

"Personal, private things that make me cringe when others can overhear."

He leaned across the table toward me. "Like what?"

"Things I love to hear when we're at home by ourselves turn me off when you say them in public."

We had a bit of a staring contest, and then he added, "What words don't you want me to say?"

Then it hit me, and I laughed. He was trying to pull me into his sexy little game. I whispered loud enough for only Drew to hear.

"Ahhhh, I see what you're doing. No way are you going to get me to say those words. Look, I'm serious. This is becoming a real problem. It's not an occasional thing now; it's becoming a habit. You can't blurt out private things when people can overhear. It's embarrassing."

His grin faded. "I think I'll go to the bathroom and have a talk with myself."

Drew got lost trying to find his way back to our table, and then he said in a frustrated tone that the soap dispenser didn't work, and the bathroom door wouldn't open. As soon as he got calmed down, the first words out of his mouth were, "Let's talk about sex."

I caught myself before rolling my eyes. "I thought you were going to have a talk with yourself about that."

Drew hung his head. "I forgot. But I'll try to do better."

Our light days are always clouded with the reality that he can't remember his good intentions from one moment to the next. He asks questions to find his way along. But the real question is this: Can I recognize and savor the humor when it comes?

February 13, 2016

Gradual, subtle things are keeping me on my toes:

- Sorting out his medicines (and mine) takes a lot more time than it used to. I have to remember to put his pills out before placing the glass of water on the table, or Drew will drink the water before I have a chance to put the medication in front of him.

- These days, everything he does takes longer, so I have to plan ahead. He can still shave and dress without assistance, but if we need to leave at a certain time, I need to give him several reminders before he gets up and going. At this point, he needs an additional half hour, and that doesn't count the extra ten minutes when he'll say, "I need to go to the bathroom," before getting into the car.

- He pushes the shopping cart for me at the grocery store but follows along behind me at a slower pace, so I have to keep looking back to make sure he's still there. I remind myself to smile and wink and otherwise send happy glances so he will feel affirmed. Too many people shop with scowls on their faces. I don't want to be one of them.

- I've learned not to place a doggy treat in Drew's hand and then turn my back because he will shove the bone-shaped biscuit into his mouth. I usually find out when he says, "This thing doesn't have much flavor."

- His peripheral vision has shrunk, so he can only see things that are right in front of him. Apparently, by the mid-term period of the disease, Alzheimer's patients have the equivalent of tunnel vision. Coupled with his hearing loss, he often doesn't know I'm there when I'm standing right beside him. When I come from the side to place his breakfast on the table, it startles him, so I've learned to touch his shoulder before putting the plate down.

- When the mailman comes, I have to make sure to listen for the mail truck so I can get to the envelopes before Drew does because he'd hide the bills.

- He's easily bored, so any random fart becomes "an event" at our house. After "an event," he will imitate the sound and then chuckle for a good ten to fifteen minutes over how funny it struck him. There's no way I can just say, "Excuse me," and have him ignore it. Nope. But this is not new, just exaggerated.

This pattern dates back to our honeymoon in Niagara Falls when we were standing alone in the parking lot of the Best Western motel. He kissed me, and I tooted softly. I didn't say a word, figuring he would dismiss it. But, nooo.

"What was that?"

And I replied, "What was what?"

"That noise."

"What noise?"

"That noise that sounded like a fart. Did you fart? You did. You farted!"

Of course, I confessed in the motel parking lot, and I am still confessing this many years later, always resulting in a good belly laugh. The difference now is that he replays "the event" ten times and is still laughing long after I have changed the subject.

February 22, 2016

What a great time we had yesterday. My brothers, Mike and Jim, and their wives, Mary and Shelly, picked us up and treated us to dinner in a private room at Nage in Rehoboth Beach. Family stories, many of them side-splitting, punctuated the gourmet meal.

My favorite is the one that Jim told us. He was working with several other coaches at the University of Delaware football camp one summer in the late '90s, and they went to dinner together at a place called "The Crab Trap." The guys hoped to get some steamed crabs and beer after a hard, hot day of coaching the players.

It turned out to be a classier place than they anticipated. The young waitress tilted her nose in the air and looked down at them as she approached the table. Her posture looked as forced as her words sounded. "Are you ready to order?"

"Do you have crabs?" one of the coaches asked.

"Crabs?" The snarly waitress's lip curled, and the scowl on her face spoke volumes even before she added, "This restaurant does *not* serve *crabs*."

The coaches were famished, so they quickly scanned the menu and placed their orders. And then they waited . . . and waited . . . for the food to come.

When the waitress returned to check on their drinks, one of the coaches asked, "Why is this restaurant called "The Crab Trap" when you don't serve crabs?"

"Well," the waitress replied, "down the street is a restaurant called "The Golden Dragon," and they don't serve dragons."

The coach raised one eyebrow and asked, "Then, do you have frog legs?"

The waitress almost smiled. "Why, yes we do!"

Without changing his expression, he spoke very matter-of-factly. "Well, if you have frog legs, why don't you just hop yourself into that kitchen and get us our food?"

There were other stories, too, and we left the restaurant still laughing, with tears streaming down our cheeks. You can see why I like to spend time with my brothers. And this was only *one* of their many stories. With full tummies and quieter conversation in the van, we arrived home refreshed, promising to get together again soon.

In a follow-up e-mail this morning, Shelly said that when she hugged Drew goodbye, she told him, "We love you," and Drew said that he loved them, too. The next words in her e-mail lit up like neon, and I will hold them close to my heart for a long time: **"If he doesn't quite know the names, he knows the love."**

February 24, 2016

Drew's sleepy eyes peered at me from beneath the covers as he gave his lazy arms a stretch. "Is this our first morning together?"

I thought I would be used to this by now—trying to see the world through his eyes. But I haven't yet captured the fullness of what it means to wake up feeling like this is the first morning of our honeymoon. I was tempted to get on with my morning routine—so many things need my attention—but I slowed myself down to embrace this romantic opportunity and think like a bride as I explained our forty-year history of waking up together. I don't know how long this phase will last before it morphs into another less enjoyable reality, so I want to make the most of it.

He's sleeping more now. It's not unusual for him to nap in the recliner for two hours after breakfast and again in the afternoon. He's usually in bed by 9:00, watches TV until 11:00, and then sleeps all night. One good thing is that his naps allow me to catch up on writing, household finances, and other things that require concentration, so I don't have to steal time in the wee hours as often as I did before.

February 27, 2016

He couldn't wait ten minutes for me to throw some clothes on. No, he was out of Cokes and needed them right away. He hasn't driven in a while, and I didn't know if he even remembered how to start the car. Sure enough, he came back in and asked me which key to use. I know he's a careful driver (it's just that he has no sense of direction), so I figured I'd let him try. Off he went. It should have taken him ten minutes to go to the 7-Eleven, but half an hour later, he got out of the car with two bags. We usually buy canned soft drinks in a box, but this time he came home with twenty-four Cokes in 16.9 oz. bottles.

"It was awful," he said. "I had to go to three stores, and the traffic on the highway was so bad, I turned around and came back in town before I found these."

"Where'd you wind up?" I asked, inspecting the bags for a clue.

"I don't know, but I'll never do that again. No more shopping for me."

The white bags didn't have a logo or any identification. But in the bottom of one was a plastic tray with Domino's on it.

That night, we went to Arena's in Georgetown for dinner and drove past Dominos. I stifled a laugh when I saw it. The whole front of the building is glass, with a big Coke machine and stacks of six-pack Coke bottles in clear view. Drew was on the hunt for Cokes, and *ta-da!* There they were in front of him, like a gift from God.

After dinner, when the waitress presented us with the bill, he looked in his wallet and asked if I had any money. I thought it was strange since I had just given him $60 that morning. But then I realized that twenty-four of those Cokes at Domino's pricing must have wiped him out.

On the way home, he leaned his head against the headrest and sighed. "I really like being chauffeured around." I hope he remembers that the next time he needs Cokes.

March 1, 2016

I'd had a busy day with my bookkeeper trying to get a handle on our taxes, and Drew had waited patiently for hours.

"Let's go out to dinner," he said as soon as she left. "Here's your coat."

"Anywhere in particular?" I asked as we got into the car.

He gave me his usual answer: "Wherever you want."

So I took off driving with no particular destination in mind. *Maybe Jimmy's Grill in Bridgeville*, I thought. But as I began thinking about what I would order at Jimmy's, fried chicken just came to mind. Although I hadn't mentioned it, I'd been thinking about Royal Farms fried chicken for about a week. Just as I was about to get in the left-hand lane at the intersection, I saw Royal Farms on the right and made a snap decision. "How about fried chicken from Royal Farms? We can take it home or eat there— they have a few tables and chairs."

By then, we were already there, so I drove in.

"What are we doing here?" he asked. "We don't need gas."

He used to be spontaneous and like surprises. I know better than to spring surprises on him now, but I really wanted that chicken. I ushered him inside the building and to the electronic pad where I punched in my order. He followed me to the counter to pay for it, mumbling, "What are you doing? I thought we were going to eat out."

A full day of going over income and expenses with the bookkeeper made me money-conscious. "This'll cost less. Did you want to eat here or take it home?"

He didn't answer, so I rounded up napkins and forks and guided him to one of three tiny metal tables by the front window. My loving pats and soothing words didn't cut it. By the time I returned from picking up our order ten steps away, he was in full scowl.

If only I had thought of it sooner, we could have discussed it, and he would have thought it was a good idea. He needs time to process things, and I didn't think of that. All I had on my mind was that "World-Famous Chicken."

"I thought we were going out to dinner," he said when I plunked the food on the table.

The aroma of the chicken made my mouth water, and I couldn't open the box fast enough. "This *is* dinner," I said with a half-smile, "and we *are* out." My lame attempt at humor came out snarly.

I placed the coleslaw and chicken in front of him, and he said, "You tricked me. Why are you doing this? I thought we were going to a nice restaurant."

By then, I had popped a juicy, tender bite of white meat into my mouth. How could I be so selfish? Didn't I see how he just needed a little tender, loving care?

"Who are you?" he said. "You seem like a different person."

What had gotten into me? What happened to my vow to maintain a peace-filled environment for him? And for me?

"You're right," I said. "I don't know what came over me. The ambiance is definitely lacking." I couldn't seem to snap out of flippant mode.

But then I looked at him—really looked at him—and remorse set in. I apologized every way I knew how, but he wasn't buying it. He had "been good" all day, and this was his reward? I had ruined what could have been a perfect evening. On top of that, I was *rude*—a characteristic I despise in myself. After all, didn't Mom always say there's no excuse for rudeness? Placing my hand on Drew's, I said, "I'm so sincerely sorry. How can I make it up to you?"

144

He pouted. "You can't. There's nothing you can do to make it right."

"Would you be up for a nice drive to Seaford for an ice cream sundae at Friendly's?"

He brightened ever so slightly. "Ice cream?" He nodded his head. "I guess that would be okay."

But he was silent during the half-hour drive, with zero response to my lighthearted jabbering. I parked in front of Friendly's, and we got out. It was hard to see his face in the twilight, so I tried to read his body language. He crossed his arms over his chest and spoke slowly. "Do you know . . . how often . . ."

Oh boy, here we go again. He would fixate on the fried chicken fiasco all night long. And then he finished his sentence.

". . . I thank God for you?"

He melted my heart right there in the parking lot.

That ice cream sundae was the most romantic dessert we ever shared. How fitting that they call it a "Happy Ending."

'Tis the little things that bug us
and tend to hold us back.
We can sit upon a mountain
but not upon a tack.

— Author Unknown

CHAPTER TWELVE

So Many Subtle Changes

March 7, 2016

Drew doesn't know we're married now. I can tell him six times in a row—or twenty—and it just doesn't stick. This afternoon, he sat attentively in a chair and said, "So, tell me all about yourself." I gave him an overview of the highlights of my life and ended with the fact that I've been married to him for more than forty years and we raised three children in this house who now have adult children of their own.

Two minutes later, he asked, "What happened to the one I've been dating?"

I wasn't sure what to say, so I came up with, "You mean, Candy?"

His face brightened. "Yes, Candy. That's the one."

When I said, "Nothing happened to her—I'm Candy," he blinked, and the look on his face was pure confusion.

I can't imagine how puzzling this must be for him.

"I'll bet you just woke up from a nap, and you're coming out of a dream." I pinched his cheek and winked. "There'd better not be anyone else. You belong to me!"

March 10, 2016

Today's subject is sex. Last September, our routine was comfortably infrequent, but lately, things have changed. Drew may have lost interest in online checker matches and reading, but his interest in sex is on his mind all the time now. It's like he's just discovered the mystery of his anatomy and now wants to exercise it.

In the entirety of our marriage, we have never refused each other when one of us hints about intimacy. But last week when he gave me a friendly look and said, "We haven't made love very often, have we?" I said, "Yes, honey. We've made love for the last three nights, and I don't think this sixty-eight-year-old body can handle it that often."

We talked it through, and he said he wanted me to enjoy it and never meant to pressure me in any way. I assured him that he satisfied me completely and I didn't feel pressured. I just didn't want us to overdo it.

"So," he said, "how many times have we had sex since we've been together?"

I reached for the calculator. "Let's see," I said. "There are fifty-two weeks in a year. If we made love once a week—sometimes it's more, sometimes less—times forty years—that would be 2,080 times."

He grinned. "Then, I guess we can skip tonight."

March 11, 2016

Tonight, Drew asked if someone has been messing with his desk.

Last December, he asked me to write the names and dates on the back of a picture of my daughter and her family so he would know who they were. He just came across it on his desk and didn't know what it was and who had put it there.

He also showed me a card with a boyhood picture of him with his dog that Kelly had made for his birthday a year ago. He recognized himself and Trixie but didn't understand why it was on his desk and where it came from. When I told him, he didn't believe me, so I said we must have a flock of fairies that bring him presents. Oddly enough, that fantasy seemed to satisfy him.

March 15, 2016

Drew's brothers, Howard and Dean, stopped by for an impromptu visit. In a follow-up e-mail, Dean said, "I am always impressed when I go to your house (even unannounced), and everything is so neat and clutter-free. How do you do that?"

I had to laugh because there's been such a big improvement in my housecleaning over last year when I didn't have the energy to pick up *anything* because of my heart issues. I have a book, *Cut the Clutter and Stow the Stuff,* that says there are four main types of clutter styles or types of individuals: The Collector, The Concealer, The Accumulator, and The Tosser. At heart, I'm a Tosser with strong Concealer tendencies—in contrast to Drew, who is an Accumulator.

Since January, when I began to feel stronger, I've been making a conscious effort to clean up one area at a time (a drawer, one closet, a pile on the floor, one stack of papers). After pulling out *EVERYTHING* and putting back only what I need, I do my best to keep it that way. Then I call my friend, Doris, who comes in and collects all the good stuff to share with her friends and grandkids. I still have a long way to go on the parts you can't see in a walk-through, but decluttering helps me think more clearly. It's nice to be able to open a cupboard and not have things fly out. Eliminating the junk is good for Drew, too, since it causes less confusion.

Here's a snippet I found in the archives at ALZinfo.org (reviewed by William J. Netzer, Ph.D., Fisher Center for Alzheimer's Research Foundation at The Rockefeller University):

> Making life easier for someone with Alzheimer's disease may mean making such simple changes as limiting household clutter, according to new research from Georgia Tech and the University of Toronto.
>
> The findings suggest that, under certain circumstances, reducing visual clutter could help people with memory problems better perform everyday tasks. For example, the researcher's note, buttons on a telephone tend to be the same size and color; only the numbers are different. These slight visual differences may make dialing a phone number especially difficult for someone with memory problems.
>
> Other research has shown that eliminating visual clutter may make life easier for someone with Alzheimer's. Furniture and carpets that have a busy pattern or that are a similar color, for example, may be difficult to distinguish for someone with dementia, making it more likely that someone would suffer from falls and broken bones, a common problem for those with Alzheimer's disease. Similarly,

plates, serving dishes, utensils, and tablecloths that are a similar color or that have busy patterns may make it harder for someone with Alzheimer's to eat a meal. Instead, choose a bold, simple color that's different for each.

Hopefully soon, Drew will give me permission to tackle his stuff. (See Appendix for more tips from ALZ.org on rummaging, hiding, and hoarding behaviors.)

March 27, 2016

Our Easter was pretty much like any other Sunday: watching John Hagee, Charles Stanley, and David Jeremiah on the TV instead of attending church and Drew dozing in front of the television most of the day. My spiritual act of worship involved delving into a publishing project while listening to praise music. We had to pass on dinner with the family because Drew can no longer handle the commotion of big crowds, so I cooked a turkey breast, broccoli and cauliflower, and redskin potatoes. At least it was easier on my diet than facing the temptation of ham, macaroni and cheese, and a table full of desserts.

I managed to bypass all of the Easter candy this year and bought myself flowers like the ones that Drew used to bring me. We talked with or saw all three kids, a friend gave me potted tulips, and we received several Easter cards—all of which made me feel connected to the outside world.

Somehow, though, being set apart from tradition has caused the resurrection message to resonate deeper in my spirit than usual. Jesus went to the cross alone. I am not alone because He is very present in our home, and the cross He has given me to bear is light.

March 30, 2016

When you're living with someone, it's easy to miss subtle changes that indicate a shift in capabilities. It wasn't that long ago when Drew could sort out socks from underwear from T-shirts, fold them, and put them away. For a while now, I've been doing it myself. Last night I asked him to empty the dryer while I continued to work on a manuscript. Imagine my shock when I found the laundry spread out piece by piece all over the kitchen. He couldn't put likes with likes, so he did what he could. Oh, how we take for granted the ability to sort and fold our clothes.

Yesterday he said, "Can you make me a sandwich? I tried, but it wore me out." I saw the culprit immediately: a new loaf of bread with a cellophane wrapping inside the plastic bag that he couldn't figure out how to open. For someone like him who has cognition problems, there are booby traps all over the house.

Like last night. He brought the bottle of CoQ10 to me and asked, "Do I use one of these in the dishwasher?" Who would have thought he would confuse a vitamin pill with a dishwasher pod? At least he senses there's something wrong and is good about asking before he does it.

Then there's the curdled milk I found in the refrigerator that he used on his cereal the night before. He used to be so keenly aware of the expiration date and always made sure the milk was fresh. Since I drink almond milk, I didn't notice how low his milk was getting. When I did, I checked the expiration date, and it was a week after the "use by" stamp. Oh, the stench and globs when I poured it down the drain! He had a new bottle right behind it with a good date but never mentioned anything about the old milk "tasting funny." I'll check it often from now on. I guess his senses of smell and taste are fading away, too. That may explain his loss of appetite.

Drew has always been safety conscious, but now he's becoming obsessive/compulsive about it. When we got up from our table in the restaurant after dinner, he blew out the candle and didn't see anything wrong with that. I winked at the waitress who saw him do it and hurried him out the door before he noticed the lit candles on all the other tables.

He's constantly unplugging things, like computers set for automatic upgrades in the wee hours, along with lamps that don't turn on the next time I try to use them. Oh, well. This is a minor inconvenience for me, but an important activity for him as protector of the castle. He needs to be needed, and he has lost control of so much of his life that surely I can allow him this small comfort.

Every night he makes his rounds throughout the house, closing blinds and locking doors. It takes about three or four times before he's content. Then, just as we're putting our heads on our pillows he'll ask, "Is the front door locked?" So I tell him, "I don't know. Why don't you check it?" and he bounces out of bed and comes back announcing that it's locked.

In the morning, I've been going around the house opening the blinds but realized I didn't need another job, so I asked him if he could do it. He said, "I thought I did," and then he paused and added, "but I guess the only thing I could really remember is if I s— my pants."

April 2, 2016

Lately, his most frequent question has changed from "How long have we been going together?" to "What's our status?" He wants so earnestly to know all about our history but no sooner do I say, "We've been married forty years" than he says, "I know what I wanted to ask you. How long have we been seeing each other?"

I smiled. "Forty years."

"How long have we been together now?"

"That would be forty years, ever since we got married."

After another three questions in quick succession, he said, "I guess the answer to everything is forty years."

"Pretty much," I said, and he immediately asked, "So, how long have we been married?"

I leaned forward, gazed at him intently, and said, "Get ready . . ."

His eyes widened, and he answered for me. "Forty years?"

So far, I haven't gotten tired of finding creative, often playful ways to answer him, but I guess I could just give a broken record response since he wouldn't know the difference. Dictionary. com's definition for a broken record is, "someone or something that annoyingly repeats itself, like a vinyl record with a scratch." Did you know that repetition without resolution is considered a method of psychological torture? So the creative answers are mostly for my benefit. The effort to find something fresh in the redundancy keeps me from feeling trapped in what could easily seem like a torture chamber.

What Drew needs most is reassurance, so I tell him, "I love you more now than when we first met." When he asks why, I say, "Because I know your heart, and you always want what's best for me." That seems to satisfy him and stalls his questions about "our status" for a good five minutes or so. The affirmation serves another purpose: it helps to anchor me in the satisfaction that comes from putting others first.

April 4, 2016

One thing that keeps me going is humor. One of my Bermuda classmates forwarded this to my inbox this afternoon. I don't know where it originated or who wrote it, but it sure spoke to me:

My goal for 2016 was to lose just 10 pounds. Only 15 to go.

Ate salad for dinner! Mostly croutons & tomatoes. Really just one big, round crouton covered with tomato sauce. And cheese. FINE, it was a pizza. I ate a pizza.

How to prepare tofu:
1. *Throw it in the trash.*
2. *Grill some meat.*

I just did a week's worth of cardio after walking into a spider web.

I don't mean to brag but . . . I finished my 14-day diet in 3 hours and 20 minutes.

A recent study has found that women who carry a little extra weight live longer than men who **mention it.**

Kids today don't know how easy they have it. When I was young, I had to walk 9 feet through shag carpet to change the TV channel.

Senility has been a smooth transition for me.

Remember back when we were kids, and every time it was below zero out they closed school?

Me neither.

I may not be that funny or athletic or good looking or smart or talented . . . I forgot where I was going with this.

I love being over 50. I learn something new every day. And forget five others.

A thief broke into my house last night. He started searching for money, so I woke up and searched with him.

My dentist told me I need a crown. I was like: I KNOW! right?

I think I'll just put an "Out of Order" sticker on my forehead and call it a day.

April 15, 2016

It's a good thing I stocked up on some humor because these past few days haven't been very much fun.

On Tuesday, I represented Drew at a family partnership meeting with his brothers but couldn't tell him anything about it. On Wednesday the three kids and I met with the elder law attorney, but I couldn't tell him anything about that either. Both times, I had to make excuses about where I was going, so I'm not only feeling guilty about keeping things from him but have the burden of facing all this heavy stuff about finances, trusts, annuities, and major life decisions. One good thing is that the family and I are bonding closer by the day.

When I came home from the meetings, instead of being able to relax and sort through the ton of information I'd been bombarded with, I had to be careful to appear "normal," whatever that is. If I don't, Drew asks Me, "What's wrong?" and then I have to come up with an answer. I know, because that's what happened.

For four or five years, we've known that the beams under the house have rotted and need to be replaced. (Drew had stopped opening the vents in the foundation, and nobody noticed.) Ten minutes before the contractor got here, Troy and I reminded Drew he was coming. Drew insisted there wasn't anything wrong with the house and asked for proof. Troy and I gave him a tour of the new cracks in the walls and the half-inch shift in the doors. Then we demonstrated for him how the china cabinet in the dining room rattles. He responded, "If it's so bad, why didn't anybody tell me about it?"

"We discussed it many times," I said, "you just don't remember," which, of course, he didn't want to hear.

Just then, Gerald rang the doorbell and, after his inspection of what needs to be done, gave Drew a gentle overview of the situation. Because the crawl space is too shallow, he'll need to approach the work from the top down, which means half of the house will be pretty well torn up (and closed off) for a couple of weeks. Fortunately, our bedroom (with TV) and the master bath is located next to the kitchen and laundry room, so we'll be able to live in that part of the house while the work is underway. Any slight change in Drew's routine jolts him (remember the nightlight?), so it's going to be a challenge, but we can't have the house falling in.

All of this is mentally and emotionally exhausting. I didn't want to have to think anymore, so I took a nap this afternoon, and the world faded away. Five minutes after I woke up—no kidding—Drew began to sing, "Make the world go away, and get it off my shoulders." I had to smile. Maybe that's God's way of showing me that Drew is still tuned into my needs.

April 16, 2016

One of the things I do for myself is participating in the monthly meeting of Delmarva Christian Writers' Fellowship. This month, Stephen Klyce serenaded us with piano music while we worked on a poetry writing exercise.

I chose haiku (the rhythm of five syllables, then seven, and closing with five) because I've never felt comfortable with that format and I wanted to stretch myself. All I could think about was Drew. Rather than strive at composing, I closed my eyes and allowed my body to relax fully for the first time in a week. I sensed the Lord's presence, and those few minutes were as refreshing to me as a week's vacation.

A phrase came into my mind—"tender heart"—so I opened my eyes and wrote it down. Other words began to flow. This is what I came up with for my haiku. One stanza for Drew, one for me, and one for us:

Tender heart, confused.
Sleeps, forgets, questions—again.
Yet, he feels my love.

Heavy weight to bear:
Household bills, doctors, and pills.
Yet, I feel his love.

Unknowns every day,
Each attempting to be kind.
Yet, we feel God's love.

April 19, 2016

This morning's question at the breakfast table was, "Why am I here?"

I knew it wasn't a rhetorical question. Placing my hand on his, I said, "You're here because this is where you live."

"Who are you?" he asked, and I simply said, "I'm your wife."

I was prepared for that, but his next question caught me off guard. "This is not where I grew up?"

I tried to take it in stride and said, "No, this is the home we've shared for the past forty years since we got married in 1975."

"So, we're married, and I'm right where I belong?"

I nodded. "Right where you belong."

Tonight, just as we were settling into bed about to go to sleep, he asked several versions of the same question: "Where are we?" "Whose house is this?" "Who owns this house?"

I assured him, "This is where we live." "It's our house." "You and I own it." And finally, "All you need to know is that you're in a safe place with someone who loves you. Go to sleep. You can look around to your heart's content in the morning."

Within a few minutes, he was sound asleep. Me? I'm wide awake.

April 20, 2016

For a while now, Drew has had difficulty understanding the difference between the recycle bin and the regular trash. More than six months ago, I went through a big explanation about paper, glass, plastic, etc. and, after a long discussion, wound up identifying the containers as "Good Trash" and "Bad Trash." I put post-it notes on the wall above them, and that worked for a while. This morning, I caught him trying to combine the two half-full containers (heaven knows how many other times he did that), so I went through the whole explanation from scratch for about the twentieth time. When I finished, he nodded and said, "So, I can just combine them, right?"

Wrong.

I took the post-it notes off the wall and said as lovingly as I could, "No, we can't combine them, hon. That's why we have two trash cans, so we can keep them separate." Poor guy—he can't even take out the trash without feeling like he's being reprimanded.

And I have one more job to do.

April 21, 2016

Drew has a new game. Now, some of you may think this is too personal and private to share, but I want this book to be an accurate depiction of the life of this married couple going through Alzheimer's together. So here it is.

He follows me around the house looking for opportunities to expose himself. Like a young boy who has just discovered his magical appendage, he's preoccupied with it and wants to show off. It's disconcerting when I'm trying to relax and suddenly there he is—in front of me with his zipper down.

I need to discourage this behavior but don't want to risk making him feel rejected. So I ooh and aah about what a beauty he has there and then turn my gaze away.

Love from the center of who you are;
don't fake it.
Run for dear life from evil;
hold on for dear life to good.
Be good friends who love deeply;
practice playing second fiddle.

— Romans 12:9-10 (MSG)

CHAPTER THIRTEEN

Coping Mechanisms and the Vibe

April 22, 2016

A friend referred me to an article in a blog entitled "16 Things I Would Want If I Got Dementia." It's a heartfelt wish list from a dementia care worker by Rachel Wonderlin:

"Rules for a Good Life"

- *If I get dementia, I want my friends and family to embrace my reality. If I think my spouse is still alive, or if I think we're visiting my parents for dinner, let me believe those things. I'll be much happier for it.*

- *If I get dementia, I don't want to be treated like a child. Talk to me like the adult that I am.*

- *If I get dementia, I still want to enjoy the things that I've always enjoyed. Help me find a way to exercise, read and visit with friends. If I get dementia, ask me to tell you a story from my past.*

- *If I get dementia, and I become agitated, take the time to figure out what is bothering me.*

- *If I get dementia, treat me the way that you would want to be treated.*

- *If I get dementia, make sure that there are plenty of snacks for me in the house. Even now, if I don't eat I get angry, and if I have dementia, I may have trouble explaining what I need.*

- *If I get dementia, don't talk about me as if I'm not in the room.*

- *If I get dementia, don't feel guilty if you cannot care for me 24 hours a day, seven days a week. It's not your fault, and you've done your best. Find someone who can help you, or choose a great new place for me to live.*

- *If I get dementia, and I live in a dementia care community, please visit me often.*

- *If I get dementia, don't act frustrated if I mix up names, events or places. Take a deep breath. It's not my fault.*

- *If I get dementia, make sure I always have my favorite music playing within earshot.*

- *If I get dementia, and I like to pick up items and carry them around, help me return those items to their original places.*

- *If I get dementia, don't exclude me from parties and family gatherings.*

- *If I get dementia, know that I still like receiving hugs or handshakes.*

- *If I get dementia, remember that I am still the person you know and love.*

April 24, 2016

The contractor is confident that the house isn't going to cave in any minute, so we're postponing the structural work until autumn (or longer). He also says he may be able to do the work from beneath the house instead of cutting up the floors and saturating the house with dust.

In the meantime, I've contacted a realtor to see if we can sell the old Bedford Motors building where Drew worked most of his life. It's in such bad shape that no insurance company will cover it. We have a tenant who pays good rent, but he's planning to retire soon. I'm hoping this can be done without having to put a "For Sale" sign in front that Drew might see when we drive by. I hate sneaking around and hiding things from him. On top of that, I'm such a bad liar.

In the middle of the night, Drew asked, "Who do I have here?" I went through my spiel of "your wife for almost forty-one years." He had other questions about where we were—the bedroom didn't look familiar to him. I think the decline is progressing even faster now, so the lying may not be necessary much longer. That's a bittersweet thought because I know that the next phase will be even more challenging.

Mom always said, "Do the best you can with what you have and trust God to get you through whatever comes." A wise woman, my mom. Oh, how I miss her. Just the sound of her voice would have comforted me, and she would have held me and let me sob until I felt cleaned out and strong again.

Strangely, I don't feel the need to sob right now. Maybe that's because the strong, invisible arms of God are holding me together as I put one foot in front of the other to face "whatever comes."

April 30, 2016

The changes are happening faster now. Drew didn't shave yesterday or the day before. He sleeps ten to twelve hours a night, gets up to eat breakfast and then naps in the recliner until lunch time. After lunch, he dozes until dinner and then gets into bed around 8:00 to watch television. I know I should get him moving, but he just wants to be left alone, and I don't seem to be able to muster up the strength to push him. There are some adult day care places with wonderful activities nearby, but since I can't get him up and moving at home, it would be futile to suggest them.

He has become apathetic and listless. He does enjoy music, so I bought him several CDs of golden oldies, and a friend even sang some songs to him in short videos that briefly brightened his day. I try to get him interested in doing even little things like emptying the dishwasher, but he goes to the bedroom instead. Until a few days ago, if I left a dirty pot in the sink with soap and hot water in it, he would finish scrubbing it and leave it for me on the counter, all clean and dry. The last two times, I stared at the pot in the morning—still in the sink—and the cold water stared back as if it were mocking me. He is losing his ability to initiate or follow through on anything.

Today I went to the grocery store and asked him to go with me, but he said he wasn't ready to get dressed. (I can relate. Sometimes I want to stay in my pajamas all day, too.) When I got home, instead of greeting me at the door to take the bags into the kitchen, he stood in the middle of the room, making it hard for me to walk around him.

He asked what he could do to help and then answered himself: "I guess I could move out of your way."

I smiled as I swung the bags onto the counter but felt like bawling, so I hurried back to the trunk for more bags before he could see my chin quiver.

He shuffles his feet, scraping the soles as he walks. He is so unsteady that I had to hold onto his arm in the parking lot a couple of days ago when we went to dinner. Last night, Buttercup needed to go out in the middle of the night, so he got up with her. I thought that was progress, but when he finished, instead of sitting down to take off his shoes, he stood in the bedroom doorway and almost fell over. Fortunately, he caught himself before hitting his head on the corner of the dresser. While watching him from the bed, I decided that from now on I need to be the one to take the dog out at night.

Yesterday and the previous day during mid-afternoon, he asked where he was. He doesn't recognize his own home and often walks around the house at night searching for something that looks familiar. At least he recognizes the backyard in the daylight.

May 5, 2016

The big disturbance tonight involved a wounded baby bunny Drew rescued from the claws of our black cat Midnight, the great hunter. As he called for me, I could tell from the sound of his voice that it was urgent, so I flew to the kitchen. There he stood, cradling a fur ball in his hands. He held a paper towel against the bunny's bleeding tummy and said, "Can you help?"

I took the bunny from him and held him gently for about a half hour, pressing the paper towel against his abdomen until the bleeding stopped. I don't know if the little guy is going to make it, but the precious bunny is lying comfortably (from what I can tell) on a hand towel in a cardboard box. I suspect there may be internal injuries, but I guess we'll find out in the morning if we have a bunny to feed—or bury.

Drew is so tenderhearted and compassionate—two of the many qualities I have always admired in him. During the recent decline in his health, it seems that this attribute of sensitivity is increasing. Even though that's a good thing, it makes me more sensitive, too.

I checked before going to bed, and the bunny is already cold to the touch. The Lord giveth, and the Lord taketh away. Blessed be the name of the Lord.

May 6, 2016

To cope with the stress that bombards me daily, I've developed the habit of listening to praise music while I work at the keyboard. Today's CD is *The Greatest Praise Songs of the Church: Jesus, Draw Me Close* by Guideposts and Maranatha.

The song playing now is "He Is Able":

> He is able, more than able,
>> To accomplish what concerns me today.
> He is able, more than able,
>> To handle anything that comes my way.
> He is able, more than able,
>> To do much more than I could ever dream.
> He is able, more than able,
>> To make me what He wants me to be.

The words are a powerful reminder that Father God is present and at work in me even when—no, *especially* when—I feel helpless in the face of my circumstances. Jesus is in this with me, strengthening me for the task at hand and the challenges yet to come. I know that the Holy Spirit is using this experience to change me more into the likeness of Christ.

For one thing, He is slowing me down and giving me a deeper appreciation for the small, intangible things of life. I'm learning to talk less and listen more. I may not feel as "productive" as before, but going through Alzheimer's with Drew serves to reorder my days, helping me to glean the wheat (the things that last) and leave the chaff (the things that have no place in eternity).

While listening to my praise CDs during the day, sometimes the melody or words of a song will stir my spirit. When that happens, I still my fingers and close my eyes. Then, almost always I am transported to a place where my soul is keenly aware of the presence of the Lord. By the time my mini-worship comes to an end, my mind, will, and emotions are refreshed, and I resume my work (or tending to Drew) with an attitude adjustment I didn't even know I needed.

My dear friend, Joyce, gave me the following poem, which I hope resonates as deeply with you as it has with me:

"Give Thanks, My Child"
by
Joyce Thomas

"In everything give thanks, My child,"
the Lord one day said to me.
"For I am worthy of your praise,
regardless of what you see."

Thus, began an adventure in life
that continued week after week,
until my attention was fully on Him
and His face alone did I seek.

First, my air conditioner froze;
then my icemaker quit.
Next, my car ran hot,
and my finances were hit.

My house was invaded by bees,
and my trusty computer broke.
My daughter wrecked her car,
and, folks, this was no joke!

Then, *my* car would suddenly die
whenever it had a notion,
and I became a sitting duck
for an accident (or painfully slow corrosion).

My clothes dryer gave up the ghost,
and the septic tank needed inspection.
I wondered what was coming next,
and my dog got an ear infection.

The problems tried to drag me down,
but the instructions were still the same:
The Lord promised His victory
if I continued to praise His Name.

By thanking Him in the midst of my mess
and letting Him take the lead,
He gave me answers I didn't have
and met my every need.

May 8, 2016

I learned something today. Recently, I've been entertaining the thought of discontinuing the newspaper because Drew rarely opens it anymore. But this afternoon, he asked me where it was. I retrieved it from the trash and said, "What do you want with this? It'll soon be tomorrow, and you'll have a new paper."

His answer gave me a new appreciation for his powers of reasoning: "Because that's how I tell what day it is."

It occurred to me that when he looks at a calendar, even if I point out the square that is "today," it must look like a puzzle to him; however, the newspaper always has only one date, the current one. I decided that the expense of the daily paper is well worth the well-being it brings to him to quietly, on his own, be able to figure out what day it is.

I could write the date and day of the week on a marker board, but then it would be another thing that Candy does for him that he can't do for himself. This way, he keeps the routine of retrieving the paper from the front yard every day, which gives him a sense of purpose, and he can check the date on his own. The expense of the daily paper is a small price to pay to guard his self-esteem.

Tonight, I learned something else. Drew came into my office for his evening quiz session. "We're not married, right?"

This time, I gave a different response than usual. "I think you know the answer," I said with a smile. "How about if you tell *me* how many years we've been married."

He frowned slightly and tentatively said, "Forty?"

I applauded.

He responded with another one of his nightly questions: "How long have you been living here?"

So, I followed my new formula of getting him to answer. "The same number of years we've been married. You try it. How long have I been living here?"

His face brightened, and he said, "Forty!"—this time, with more confidence.

Ten minutes later, he came back and asked, "Are you going home tonight?"

Sigh. My successful formula was short-lived. That's not a question that can be answered with, "Forty."

May 10, 2016

We went to the Southern Grille of Ellendale for dinner, and the place was packed. Drew chose a booth by the window near the entrance where waitresses hustled and bustled around us, customers flowed through the doorway, dishes clattered, and happy sounds of laughter floated in the air. Just as I began to be concerned that it might feel like chaos to him, he opened his mouth and belted out a song at the top of his lungs.

"Jesus loves meeee, this I knowwww . . . for the Biiiible tells me soooo . . ."

Now, to understand how momentous this is, you need to know that he's very reserved—a true introvert—and, until recently, never even sang at home.

I glanced around to see if anyone was looking at us, and they were all chatting as if nothing had happened.

"Little ones to Him belong," I said, reaching for his hand. "They are weak, but He is strong."

Instead of resuming his loud solo, he repeated those two lines as softly as I had said them.

I'll never know why he sang "Jesus Loves Me" with such gusto. Maybe to center himself and regain control in the midst of all the hubbub. Then our soup arrived, and whatever the reason, he stayed calm throughout dinner in spite of the commotion around us.

May 11, 2016

I've already told you I'm a bad liar, but I'm an even worse car thief.

For a long time, I've known we needed to sell our 2009 Pontiac Vibe that's been sitting idle in the driveway for nine months. Every time I proposed the idea to Drew, though, he wouldn't hear of it. After all, he "might need it" if I went somewhere in the Cadillac. But that's just the point. I don't want the car sitting there tempting him to drive.

Lately, Drew has been asking, "Do you have a car?" and "What do you drive?" I decided I could claim that the Vibe is mine and tell him it's in the shop if he asks. That's better than confessing I'm conniving with my son-in-law to steal the car so I can sell it, right?

Yesterday, Wyatt and I devised a plan to make the car disappear:

We would do it in the morning while Drew was sleeping. I would get up at 7:30 and move the Cadillac out of the driveway so Wyatt could have easy access to the Vibe. He has both sets of keys, and his dad would drop him off at our house at 7:45. Wyatt would quietly drive the car away, and I would put the Cadillac back in the driveway. It seemed like a good plan.

Last night, I set the alarm for 7:30 a.m. but woke up in the wee hours thinking I'd better turn it off so the *beep-beep-beep* didn't wake Drew. Afraid I would oversleep, I got up at 3:30, worked in my office until 7:30, and then moved the Cadillac onto the street.

This is good, I thought. *I'm getting some work done, undisturbed, and we're right on schedule.*

At 7:33, my cell phone rang. It was Wyatt telling me that he was here but the car wouldn't start—dead battery. "Do you have any jumper cables?"

So I dashed outside wearing my PJs and flip-flops, and the search began. No jumper cables in the Vibe. Maybe in the shed? We walked to the backyard, and both shed doors were locked. Troy told me a while ago where to find the key, but I couldn't remember.

"I don't know," I said. "Let's try the trunk of the Cadillac." Voila! The zippered emergency kit contained jumper cables.

I eased the Cadillac onto the grass next to the driveway and parked beside the Vibe—right by the bedroom window where Drew was sleeping—and hoped that the sound of the engine wouldn't wake him. I got out and gently closed the car door, clutching the "smart key" in my hand.

Beepity-beep! That stupid horn! The Cadillac must not like the driver to walk away with the key while the car is running. At least it only *beepity-beeped* once.

Wyatt set to work hooking up the cables. The minute he clamped them onto the Vibe, the horn started beeping, LOUD—again, and again, and again! No, we don't need the security alarm. We got it stopped.

And then Wyatt said, "Nothing's happening." There was no energy flow. "There should be sparks." So he disconnected the cables and flicked them together. Sparks galore. Yay! We were in business.

But when he reconnected them, the Vibe security alarm went off with continuous horn blasts: *BEEEEP. BEEEEP. BEEEEP. BEEEEP. BEEEEP.* Right outside Drew's bedroom window. *BEEEEP. BEEEEP. BEEEEP. BEEEEP.*

Wyatt couldn't disconnect the cables, or the battery wouldn't charge. *BEEEEP. BEEEEP. BEEEEP.* He grabbed the Vibe key fob and pressed the red button.

The horn finally stopped. *Praise the Lord!*

I raced into the house with my flip-flops flopping and my PJs flapping and then slowed to a stroll as I entered the bedroom to check on Drew. He was still in bed but stirring. "What's all the noise?" he wanted to know. I told him it was just a car at the apartments across the street, and he said, "Sounded like it was right in our yard."

Duh.

So I chitchatted with him about what a nice day it looked like it was going to be. "Do you want me to turn on the TV?" I asked, hoping the sound of it would drown out future beeping. "Would you like some coffee or do you want to sleep a little longer?"

He said if I wanted to watch TV that would be fine. He didn't want coffee and thought he would sleep some more. I sat in the recliner next to the bed for a couple of minutes, pretending to watch the news while my mind raced about how I could sneak outside to help Wyatt with the jumper cable challenge.

When Drew looked like he was dozing off, I slipped out the front door.

During that time, Wyatt had finished charging the battery, moved the Vibe to the street, and parked the Cadillac back in the driveway.

We laughed and said we'd be talking about this for years. After giving him a quick hug, I hotfooted it into the house—and almost ran smack into Drew, who was standing in the living room.

"Who was that?" he wanted to know.

Trepidation sizzled through me. He had looked out the window and caught me hugging another man.

"Um, it was Wyatt. He had the day off and was in the area."

"Oh," he said, and I held my breath for what might follow. "That's nice. What's for breakfast?"

Fast forward to 6:30 tonight.

Kim said that Wyatt sent her a text saying he couldn't wait to tell her about the hilarious morning we had. She teaches and had to wait for her break before she could talk with him, so the suspense was building. When she called back and got the scoop, she thought the story was so funny that she shared it with a co-worker. And—

guess what? The co-worker and her husband came to test drive the Vibe after work and sent me an e-mail saying they can have a check ready tomorrow and meet me at the DMV. SOLD! Whoever heard of a car selling in less than ten hours without the owner having to say a word? Sounds like a God-thing to me.

Drew didn't notice that the car was missing until tonight. I told him it had a dead battery and was in the shop getting an overhaul. Five minutes later, he asked again, "Where's the other car?" Next time, he might ask which shop the Vibe is in or how long it will take to get fixed. I don't know what I'll say about that, and I can only stall so long.

But what if Drew wants to see the car? Kim and Wyatt suggested that I tell him that we're letting Kade use it since he's turning sixteen (and he will always be at golf, Little League, or doing something). I did suggest that to Drew a while back because we did the same thing with our other grandson, Trevor, years ago (so there's a smidgen of truth to that).

The leader of our support group tells us not to lie but to bend the truth. I have often bent the truth so far it's about to break, but my motivation always springs from my desire to let Drew stay in his comfortable place of denial so he doesn't have to confront the devastating reality that he has Alzheimer's. Now I've set myself up to be caught in a series of lies, which is the *worst* thing of all because I need him always to trust me. It worries me that I'm becoming so proficient at fibbing, but in the big picture of my list of things to worry about, this ranks pretty low. I'm praying that he'll forget about the Vibe. Who would have thought I'd ever want him to forget? It wasn't that long ago I was asking the Lord to help him remember.

May 13, 2016

I never know what Drew is going to say in public. Tonight, after I told the waitress that I would have soup and half a sandwich, she turned to Drew for his order. He said with an ornery grin and a weird accent, "I just came in from China, and I don't speak English." She cracked up.

After he told her he would have the same thing I ordered, she left, still smiling. And I said, still laughing, "What you said was so funny."

He gave me a blank stare. "What did I say?"

"You said, 'I just came in from China, and I can't speak English.'"

He cocked his head. "I said that?"

May 16, 2016

I think the Vibe situation is under control. For the past few days, whenever he asks when the car will be back, I've been saying that it's not coming back because we're loaning it to Kade since he's turning sixteen soon. Drew's reasoning powers have been kicking in because now he says we should put the car in Kim and Wyatt's name so their insurance instead of ours will cover it. Today I told him that was a great idea, and I'd be happy to take care of that. So, he's on board with the car not returning to our driveway. Hallelujah! What a relief that we've resolved this sticky issue together. It almost felt like old times as the two of us worked out a plan together.

Now, the question is whether or not he'll remember what we've decided. Either way, though, I'm convinced that God has answered my cry for help.

On another subject, he's been chanting, "Eenie meenie miney mo, catch a bullfrog by the toe. If he hollers, let him go" at home, in the car, and during a lull in conversation over dinner in a restaurant. It's as if he has a need to fill the silence with something, and this has become his default dialogue. He said it again today. When he finished, he smiled and added, "That's a song I just made up." Alzheimer's patients are exempt from plagiarism, right?

He's also developed the habit of forcing a burp until it sounds like a loud, obnoxious belch (a flashback of my brothers when we were kids). I give Drew a disapproving look when he does that, and then he says, "What about the laugh I got out of you?"

To this I say, "That wasn't me. That was *you* you heard laughing."

"Well," he says with a pout, "you won't catch me doing that again."

Bet I will, too, catch you doing that again.

I have learned
that life is like a roll of toilet paper.
The closer it gets to the end, the faster it goes.

— Andy Rooney

CHAPTER FOURTEEN

Intimacy

May 18, 2016

One of the most tortuous things about Alzheimer's is the repetition. You hear people say, "They repeat themselves constantly," but until you live with it, you can't know how difficult this is. Today, while I fixed his breakfast and laid out his morning pills, I counted twenty-three times in a row that Drew asked, "So, how many years have we been going together?" Twenty-three times, I answered, "We've been married forty years—almost forty-one," between bites of my breakfast.

It's like the drip, drip, drip of water, and you can't turn the spigot off. One of the ways I cope is by reminding myself that I'm doing this "as unto the Lord." Would I snap at Jesus or roll my eyes if He repeated Himself twenty-three times in a row?

Maybe the Lord is testing my patience. If so, is my reaction pleasing to Him? Maybe this isn't about me at all. Maybe enduring the day-in and day-out repetition is part of the way *I get to* love Drew . . . and Jesus.

I should be happy that Drew is pleased to be with me and that he's trying so hard to piece this mystery of our relationship together. He's cheerful and compliant, not berating and resistant. So today I'm conducting a gratitude exercise of how blessed I am to have him and the family I married into.

I *am* scheduling time for myself a minimum of once a week (lunch with a girlfriend), which gives me a break from the non-stop questions, and I get daily encouragement from family and friends through e-mails, phone calls, and cards.

Oddly enough, the responsibility of paying bills and doing all of the other household things that Drew used to handle has morphed from being a burden into a welcome distraction. When his questions threaten to overtake me, I simply say, "Hon, I have to work on taxes; do you want to help?" and he disappears into the other room.

May 30, 2016

We had a heavy downpour this morning, but the sun was still shining as Drew and I sat at the kitchen table. He was quiet, and I thought that he might begin the conversation at any moment with his usual question about how long we've been going together.

Instead, he began a different dialogue.

"Jesus, this is Drew. I wanted to tell You that the rain is beautiful. You really did a good job with this one, and I just wanted to thank You for the weather."

He paused, with a faraway look in his eyes. And then he lowered his voice an octave and said, "Thank you, Drew. I appreciate that. It's rare that someone notices and tells Me about it."

Then, he wiped tears from his eyes.

And so did I.

I shared this with my friend, Pam, and she replied in an e-mail, "Such a clear answer to my prayers, Candy. I've been praying for you—but I've also been praying for Drew. That he would have peace and joy. That he would feel loved and safe with you. That he would not forget the Lord."

In her next e-mail, she said, "I've also been praying that Drew would not forget you and his love for you."

Those prayers are being answered, too. He sometimes asks, "Where's Candy?" And when I tell him "I'm Candy," he always looks confused and then delighted. When that happens, I tell him, "You may not remember who I am, but you know you love me."

June 3, 2016

Sex is continually on Drew's mind now. For the past few months, his favorite question from morning to night has been, "Can you get pregnant?"

"No," I said.

And he wanted to know why.

So, I launched into my spiel: "I almost died after giving birth to Kim, so I had my tubes tied before we met. We've never had to think about birth control."

"What does that mean—'had your tubes tied'?"

I gave him a quick biology lesson, and he looks confused. Too much information. So I said, "It's complicated."

But he pressed again.

"I can't get pregnant," I added, "because I'm too old."

"How old do you have to be not to get pregnant?"

"After menopause, when a woman goes twelve months without a period, she can't get pregnant."

"And you've gone twelve months?"

I raised one eyebrow and smiled. "I've gone fifteen *years* without a period. Do you think that's long enough to be safe?"

He stood up, and I thought that maybe, for once, he understood. And then he said, "Do I need to wear a rubber?"

"No, hon." I smiled so he wouldn't see me gritting my teeth. "We've never had to use a condom during almost forty-one years of marriage, and there's no reason to start now."

"You mean we don't need to use these?" He held out his hand with three shiny blue packets balanced on his palm.

My eyes bulged. "Where did you get *those?*"

"In my dresser drawer," he said with the innocence of a child.

Visions of his first wife flashed before my eyes, and I grabbed them out of his hand. "These belong in the trash! If they're more than forty years old, they're dry-rotted."

Drew frowned slightly and then gave me an ornery smile. "I have more in my drawer. Should I put one on?"

June 7, 2016

My friend, Elizabeth, said she was thinking about me when she wrote this and was led to give it to me today. Little did she know it's my birthday. Her words are profound, and I receive them as a gift. I hope you will, too:

"What Is Truth?"
by
Elizabeth Boerner

For a friend to know her truth is to know herself truly. The truth is not going to look the same to everyone. For her, the truth is to move ahead into the steps that God has ordained her to take.

The truth to her is to make believe to him that his reality is the truth. Is this a life of a lie? No, simply the life of someone who is in love with the man she fell in love with so, so long ago. His truth is that everything is the same as it ever was. The same of themselves. The essence of who he has been with himself for all the days he has lived so far. How are these moments the ones that he still remembers? Why are these the chosen ones?

Does he remember his favorite color? Her favorite color? The simplest things are the most extraordinary, that is why we have to pay such close attention. The simplest things in our lives might end up being our every day. Our round and round. And we, too, might not understand why our truth doesn't make sense to others.

Today the sun is shining, yet the memory of the sunshine might go away completely when there is rain. The snow might be the first snow we have ever seen, when our truth is made of the simple things.

When does the memory fade? What can we do to stop this madness? Maybe it is all in God's grand scheme of things, preparation for the eternal.

What shall my friend do? What kind of life is this? The life of a whole person helping out the man she loves most in all the world so together they can make it another day, another hour, another minute, another second, another breath.

What shall her love do in his every day? Get through the best that he knows how without thinking about it for one moment.

How beautiful life would be without having to think about it for one moment, to simply exist and to enjoy the one that you have loved for the majority of your life.

To simply love and to be loved.

Isn't that why we are here?

June 15, 2016

Let's talk about impatience—his and mine. My subconscious is always aware of what I learned from the support group about managing agitation with someone who has Alzheimer's: Do not raise your voice or show alarm or offense; do not corner, crowd, restrain, criticize, ignore or argue with the person. In my efforts to keep him calm, however, I might have inadvertently trained him that he can always get his way.

Little by little over the past couple of years, Drew has developed the habit of making everything *urgent*—whenever he needs (wants) something, I have to jump up and do it right *now*. If I don't, he gets impatient with me, which makes me impatient with him, and we both wind up agitated. I have to bite my tongue and remind myself not to snap at him.

This began gradually but has accelerated to such a level that I'm forced to deal with the unhealthy pattern. It's a subtle form of enabling or co-dependence. He needs me, and I need to be needed—but this "jump when he says so" has gotten out of hand.

If I'm going to be an effective caregiver, allowing dysfunctional behavior on his part is not an option.

When I realized that my knee-jerk reaction in giving him instant gratification was promoting and enabling his demanding behavior, I decided to retrain him. This is not easy, let me tell you.

I began by saying, "I'll get to that in just a minute," which makes him feel he's been heard and helps him learn to wait—well, for a nanosecond, at least. But a nanosecond is long enough for me to unhook the puppet strings and be able to respond because I *want to*, not because he *tells me to.* Lately, I've been giving him a book or magazine to look at while he waits, and by the time he has flipped a few pages, the "urgent" thing isn't so urgent anymore. He's forgotten. Hey, there are some advantages to his short-term memory loss.

Recently, I read that impatience is a sign that your needs aren't being met. Certainly, Drew's needs aren't being met because he's unable to follow through on whatever he wants to do, and his solution is to ask me to do it for him "right now."

But what does my impatience reveal about my unmet needs? I came to the conclusion that whenever I get impatient, it has to do with my unmet expectations of Drew about things that he used to do (or that people do naturally) that he can't do now, like picking up after himself.

If I don't give myself a reality check on Drew's diminishing capabilities, then my cycle of impatience, guilt for overreacting, and impatience again will only spiral out of control and make us both miserable.

Some people murmur self-talk statements such as, "I guess I'm just a failure," or "I knew I couldn't handle this." In fact, this is a huge challenge even for seasoned caregivers or the most compassionate saint. It's hard. It's a testing of our mettle and a refining of our character. If we stop beating ourselves up and look for the humor, today can be a good day no matter how many times we're asked (or told) to do something we don't want to do.

I'm trying to let each grunt serve as an internal alarm, reminding me to lean on God instead of Drew and to . . . breathe in and . . . breathe out. This mini-break gives me an instant paradigm shift in which the negative feelings are replaced by the clear sense of peace described in Philippians 4:7 (NASB): "And the peace of God, which surpasses all comprehension, will guard your hearts and your minds in Christ Jesus."

Even if Drew interrupts me while I'm in the midst of my "attitude adjustment," I can respond to him with more patience and understanding than before.

June 16, 2016

While I was out having lunch with a couple of girlfriends, the gal from the attorney's office called the house and Drew answered. He just got off the phone when I came in the door and was all upset over why somebody would be calling about our deed.

"What's this about? We've got to get this straightened out. You have to call her back right away."

I figured she was just calling to clarify something and didn't realize Drew had Alzheimer's. My answers were pretty much incoherent as I spouted out whatever words came to mind, which only generated more questions. Drew's quizzing continued as he followed me down the hallway to my office. "I thought our deeds were fine. What's going on? Why would somebody be messing with our deeds?"

"Just calm down and have a seat," I said. "I'll give her a call."

But, of course, I didn't want to talk to her with *him* in the room, so I picked up the phone, turned my back to him, pressed "off" instead of "talk," and dialed some random numbers. The test of my acting skills began.

"Yes. Hello, this is Candy Abbott returning Erika's call." Short pause. "Okay, thanks. I'll hold." Pause again for an appropriate amount of time. "Yes, voice mail will be fine." Pause long enough to pretend to listen to a recorded message. "Hello, Erika, this is Candy Abbott returning your call. Sorry to miss your call earlier. I'll be leaving in a few minutes, so you can reach me on my cell phone."

I turned back to Drew and said, "She's not in but will call back."

So he sat in my office and waited for the call that's not going to come.

I began typing on a project and eventually he said, "I'll be in the bedroom watching TV."

Being deceptive is hard work, but I can live with myself because it's all for his benefit.

June 20, 2016

Tonight had to be a record for the number of times Drew wanted me to explain our lovemaking routine. He didn't want to "do it" right then, but rather just talk about it. So I went through our whole pattern and no sooner finished than—guess what?—he wanted to know again. So I explained again. And a few minutes later, and a few minutes later, and a few minutes later.

The next time, I said, "I've just spelled out our lovemaking routine in detail seven times. If I tell you again, this will be the eighth."

"But this time," he said, "I'll pay attention."

"That's what you said last time."

I had a thought. "How about if I record the details of our healthy sex life, and you can play it back whenever you want?"

"We wouldn't want a tape like that laying around. Somebody might find it."

I sighed. "You're right." And I went silent.

"Why won't you tell me? I just want to know." He pouted. No kidding, his bottom lip stuck out as if he were a child. "How do I please you? Just tell me that part."

"Okay, sexy," I said to my eighty-year-old husband. "Come with me, and I'll show you."

June 22, 2016

I lost Drew today. When I awoke from an afternoon nap in my recliner, he wasn't in his matching recliner on the other side of the bedroom where he had been dozing when I closed my eyes.

I looked in every room of the house. No Drew.

He must be taking a walk, I decided, so I returned a phone call to Wilma, who wanted to stop by and pick something up. I stapled some papers and went to the attic to get a bag for her stuff. When I had everything ready, I looked in the backyard expecting to see Drew coming toward the house. He wasn't.

A walk around the block usually takes him about fifteen minutes. It had been longer than that, and I didn't know how much *more* time had elapsed since he left before I woke up. It was a hot day, 85°, and his once strong legs now leave him unsteady. My heart lunged, and I tried to wipe the picture out of my mind of him collapsed on the street.

At the very moment I decided I needed to go looking for him, Wilma drove up. Her husband also had Alzheimer's (she's the one who helped me connect with the support group), so I knew she had experience with this sort of thing.

I greeted her with panic in my eyes. "I can't find Drew."

"Well, come on," she said, "we'll go look for him."

I handed Wilma the bag so she could put it in her car while I went to the kitchen to write, "Looking for you" on the marker board. Then we jumped into my car, and I drove around the block where Drew normally walks.

"Slow down," Wilma said as she looked into backyards and unlikely places. But I didn't slow down. I wanted to get to the next corner so I could look both ways to see Drew in his blue shirt and jeans, strolling along the street.

"Maybe he went to his brother's house," I said as I changed direction. I parked in front of Howard and Kelly's and knocked on the door while Wilma waited in the car. Nobody home.

As I drove back toward our house, it occurred to me that Drew might be looking for Buttercup. I had taken her to the groomer that morning, and he wouldn't have remembered that. *He must be in a panic.* Wilma and I retraced the same streets and expanded our search to include others in the area. Nothing.

While we were driving, I said, "This reminds me of when Kim was little. She was waiting for her daddy to pick her up, but when he got here, we couldn't find her." The panic I choked on back then when she was five was suddenly gripping me again. "But we had a happy ending," I said. "We found her sound asleep in bed, buried under the covers." Wilma and I laughed, and she said, "Maybe you should check the shed."

"Good idea," I said and soon pulled into our driveway.

While Wilma again waited in the car, praying quietly, I hurried to the backyard and toward the shed. I could see from the brick walkway that the padlock was securely fastened on the door, so I trudged up the steps of the deck, opened the sliding glass door, and checked our end of the house once more. Drew wasn't in the bathroom, and he wasn't in his recliner. And then my own words echoed in my ears, *asleep in bed, buried under the covers.*

Could it be? There *was* a slight bulge on Drew's side of the bed. I tiptoed closer, and sure enough, there he was, sleeping soundly beneath those covers.

I scampered out the front door with a grin on my face to tell my friend the good news. "I'm so glad you were here with me, Wilma. I would have been searching in full panic mode without you."

Back in the house, I erased the marker board. Drew will never know.

June 24, 2016

Guess what? Drew still has one condom in his drawer. At least tonight I got him to admit that we didn't need it, and he even agreed to dispose of it. So now the issue is *how*. Who can explain the reasoning of the Alzheimer's thought process?

"Just throw it in the trash," I said unceremoniously.

"No. Someone might find it."

"What? You think someone is going to look through our trash?"

"Yes. You'd be surprised how many people go through other people's trash."

"So you think they'll be going through our trash can looking for a condom in a foil packet that's more than forty years old?"

"Not our trash," he said. "The trash at the dump." He carried the discussion for a good ten minutes about how the garbage truck collects the trash and it winds up in the landfill. According to his perspective, there are people who sneak into the dump after dark with flashlights and go through the piles looking for treasures.

"And this little foil packet is the kind of treasure they're looking for?"

"Yes."

"Okay, then. How about if we cut it into six little pieces and toss it in the trash? They'll never find it then." I thought he would go for it.

"I have a better idea. I'll burn it."

"Burn it? You'll stink up the whole house. Do you know how bad burning rubber smells?"

"I'll burn it outside."

"I don't think you can burn things in town without a permit. Do you want me to go to the town hall and apply for a permit so you can burn your rubber in our back yard?"

"I don't want a permit. It's nobody's business that we have a rubber."

"Then don't burn it. Let me cut it up and put it in the trash."

"No," he said. And then his face brightened. "I know what. I'll bury it."

"Bury it? What if Buttercup digs it up and gets choked on it? You don't want to bury it."

"You're right," he said. "Don't worry about it. I'll take care of it." And he left the room with slumped shoulders as if he carried the weight of the world.

I didn't dare ask how he'd get rid of it.

June 25, 2016

A couple of days ago, Troy was walking his Pomeranian, Alba, in front of our house as Drew and I stepped down from the porch on our way to dinner.

"Hey, Dad. How're you doing?" Troy said.

Drew looked at him standing there at the end of our sidewalk but didn't answer, and I thought he must not have heard him.

"Anything I can do for you, Dad?"

This time, Drew said, "What?"

Troy smiled. "Do you need anything? Is there something I can do for you?"

Drew appeared puzzled and pleasantly answered as he would to a stranger, "No, but it's nice of you to offer." As he and I moved on toward the car, he said to me, "Who was that?"

Until now, he has always recognized his own son.

I found out later that there was another incident earlier that same day when Troy realized his dad didn't know him. It hit Troy hard, like a punch to the gut. He told me his mind knew about the disease and what's going on with his dad, but this was different. This hit him in the heart, and all he could think was, *I'm losing my dad.*

I live with this day in and day out, so I didn't think much about it except as a hint that we're approaching another level of decline. When Troy and I talked, I told him, "It's one thing to hear about this happening to someone else . . . and another thing entirely when it happens to *you*." I'll always remember how hard it was for me the first time Drew looked me in the eye and asked, "Where's Candy?"

194

Troy tried to describe the devastation he was feeling, and the best he could tell me was that he felt *helpless*—the perfect word for something that can't be fixed. The emotional turmoil showed up in his dreams with scenes that showed his dad here and then gone, here again and gone again.

"This really messes with your head." Troy looked at me with sad eyes that said he understood what I've been going through. "I want you to know you can count on me. The way I see it, my full-time job now is to help you and Dad as much as I can."

Never have his words meant so much.

The truth is, even if you have sown in love and faith, nobody in an Alzheimer's family escapes unscathed. But you can come through this experience stronger and more closely knit as a family.

The test of fairness
is how fair you are to those who are not.

— Malcolm S. Forbes

CHAPTER FIFTEEN

The "Driving" Discussion

June 29, 2016

Two days ago, I took Drew to the drugstore where we picked out anniversary cards for one another in preparation for our big day today—forty-one years of marriage. He kept asking me to look at each card as he considered it. "Do you like this one?" When we got home, I had to keep track of where he put it so I could help him find it this morning.

Last night, as we were about to fall asleep, Drew said, "I'm having trouble with your first name."

So I offered, "Candy."

"Don't I have a daughter named Candy?" (That's a new one.)

"No, I'm your wife, hon. You have a daughter named Dana."

In an affectionate, solemn voice, he repeated it. "Dana."

I knew that today's anniversary would bring more heartache than celebration, so I prayed last night as I dozed off that God would give me an extra measure of grace to suspend my expectations and find joy in having him here with me.

As soon as Drew woke up, he started talking about sex. *Well, I* thought, *let the honeymoon continue.* I told him that today is our anniversary, forty-one years. It only took seven times of repeating that statement before it seemed to stick.

"I need to get you a card," he said.

I was happy to help him find it on his desk. When he went to sign it, he asked how to spell his name. And then he spent a lot of time looking at the envelope. "How do you spell your name?" This time, I'm saving the envelope as well as the card because I know how diligently he labored to print every letter of my name.

I suggested that we go to Lewes and take the ferry to Cape May, New Jersey, to have lunch there, but he nixed the idea. So I proposed strolling around St. Michael's, Maryland, but he said it would be too hot. In an e-mail exchange with my friend, Betty, about what we might do, she said, "I guess you're making 80% of the decisions now." But I think we've reached the 100% mark since Drew makes no decisions now. He either declines or says, "Whatever you want."

So, in the afternoon, we both took naps in our recliners and awoke to a surprise visit from Kim, Wyatt, Kade, and Saige.

When it came time to go to dinner, I thought about the Cambridge Hyatt, but I didn't feel like driving that far. So we wound up at the LongHorn Steakhouse in Salisbury, and I used a gift card from Christmas. It was lovely. They had a picture on the wall that Drew said reminded him of his dad, so I captured it on my cell phone. At least that afforded me something memorable for our special day. In reality, all that truly matters is being together and in harmony. Tonight he knows me, and for that I am grateful.

July 8, 2016

Last week Drew's older brother came by for a visit and spent time with him in the kitchen while I met with a client in my office. When Howard got home, he told Kelly the visit hit him pretty hard—that he didn't realize how much Drew's memory had changed. "He can't remember from one minute to the next what he said."

This is heartbreaking for him and a reality check for me. The changes creep in so slowly, like an itsy-bitsy spider, that I didn't realize he had eased down to another rung of the ever-declining ladder.

About once a week for the past several weeks, Drew has asked during the night, "Where's the bathroom?" I'm tempted to say, "Right where it's always been," but that wouldn't help him. Fortunately, so far he's been able to figure it out on his own, so I didn't need to get up and guide him. I wonder how long we'll have before I have to do that . . . and more.

The day when I'll require in-home assistance may be coming soon. At this point, I have to remind him to shave after three days. He is still not ready for "strangers," but the plan is to tell him that whoever comes is a "nurse." I think that's something he could accept.

While I was visiting Kim and Wyatt this afternoon, Troy called. "Dad wants to take the truck and go for a ride. He seemed upset that the truck wasn't here—I was only gone for a few minutes. What should I do?"

This goes back to the Vibe. Almost every night when Drew is making his rounds in the house to check the doors and close the blinds, he'll look out the window and see only one car in the driveway. He asks, "Do you have a car?" and I tell him that I gave mine to Kade. "You and I share the Cadillac, and you also have the truck if you need to go somewhere when I'm gone."

Today it looks like he called my bluff.

I suggested that Troy let him drive but ask if he could ride along (maybe because he needed a few things from the store). That way, he could see firsthand if his dad's driving is safe. Whenever I ask Drew if he wants to drive, he always says, "No, you drive. I like being chauffeured around." I hoped Troy would get a similar response.

When I got home, I was relieved to see the truck in the backyard and Drew watching TV as usual in his recliner in the bedroom. He greeted me cheerfully with no mention of going for a ride in the truck.

Troy told me, "I asked him if he felt like going to the store so we could spend some father-son time together, and he said, 'Naaaa, not today.' Then I went into the shed and prayed." Later, he gave me this gentle admonishment in a text message:

> I will always try my very best to let my dad have warm and peaceful thoughts that things are the same so he will stay happy as much as possible. Taking into consideration the slow, continued decline of Dad's health over the last few months, I think it would be wise medically, and for his safety, if Dad did not drive anymore. It has nothing to do with the Cadillac or the truck. I feel this way because I love my Dad, and I love you and don't want anything to happen to either of you guys. So I will do my best, but we need to make smart decisions for Dad because if we were sick, Dad would want the same safety and care for us. Love, Troy

During our last visit with Dr. Edelsohn, he took me aside and said, "When you notice he shouldn't be driving, don't try to handle that yourself. Let me do it." It's apparent that now is the time, but Dr. Edelsohn has retired. But we're scheduled to see the new neurologist, Dr. Kemp, in nine days, and I'm going to include this note when I fill out the paperwork:

> Drew doesn't know that he has Alzheimer's and thinks that his memory problems are from the meningioma he had removed in 2013. He may or may not be ready to know the truth.
>
> The family has agreed that it is no longer safe for him to drive. Can you help with this?

July 14, 2016

Drew needed to endorse a check made out to Andrew, but he didn't think he could do it. "I only know how to write Drew," he said. I assured him that he could and spelled out each letter as he wrote A-n-d-r-e-w until he got it written.

I found a pair of his briefs folded neatly in the medicine cabinet today. When I mentioned it to him, he said, "I guess I'm losing it." I told him life is more interesting this way.

I've become accustomed to handling things that Drew used to do, such as making deposits, paying bills, getting the car serviced, and running errands. Most days, I'm able to keep things flowing.

But today my spinning top wobbled and fell off its axis when I discovered that the insurance policy I thought I canceled in April is still active. The company has continued to make automatic deductions (May, June, and July). I thought I had it resolved last month when I closed the checking account. Not so. I had to go in town and sit down with a banker who voided the overdraft fees but said I would need to contact the insurance company—which I thought I already had. And they won't return my phone calls or e-mails, so how do I get them to STOP taking my money and process a refund?

This tension, coupled with Drew's incessant questions and inability to comprehend anything I say for longer than fifteen seconds, has me wishing I could run away. But running from problems never solved them, so I spent some time breathing in . . . breathing out . . . and listening to the praise music on my computer.

And then, just when I needed it most, Elizabeth stopped by with her sunny disposition and uplifting conversation about the tangible things the Lord is doing to build up my publishing company. As always, when she left, I felt better.

And now, I wait for tomorrow to come so I can appeal to the next level of management at the insurance company . . . while Drew asks me if I'll be staying the night and sleeping in his bed.

July 18, 2016

Today is our first appointment with the new neurologist, Dr. Kemp.

The doctor reviewed Drew's previous MRIs and handled the discussion well.

Drew scored 21 out of 30 on the MMSE (Mini–Mental State Examination), which indicates a mild degree of impairment described as "Significant effect. May require some supervision, support, and assistance." (A score of 20 to 10 would put him in the Moderate category, which means we're approaching, "Clear impairment. May require 24-hour supervision.")

As gently as he could, the doctor said his score indicates that he shouldn't be driving.

"I'm an excellent driver," Drew insisted several times. Visions of Dustin Hoffman in *Rain Man* kept flashing through my mind.

Dr. Kemp gave Drew the option of scheduling someone to ride with him, evaluate his driving, and submit their report (yes or no) to the DMV about his ability to drive. But he didn't warm to that idea. Dr. Kemp ended the session by saying that he would send his notes to our primary care physician and then we should talk it over with Dr. Palekar. I'm hoping that will go well because Drew has a great deal of respect for him. I'm prepared to focus on how safety-conscious Drew has always been and appeal to him from that angle.

And so, we've had our first discussion about driving. Truthfully, I don't know what difference it will make because when he decides he wants to drive, he won't remember that he's not supposed to. When we left the office, Drew was agitated about the "bad doctor's visit." I'll just continue to drive him anywhere he wants to go.

The doctor prescribed Namenda for him. Drew said he didn't need any more pills, but I communicated with a silent nod that he *did*. At checkout, the nurse confirmed that they would call it into the pharmacy.

Drew continued to grumble as we left the doctor's office. "That's the worst doctor's appointment I ever had."

As we got in the car, I agreed with him that it certainly didn't seem fair and then kept quiet as I drove around the corner to the Atlantic Hotel, where we had lunch. I chatted about the menu choices and directed his attention to things around us (the flowers on the table, the view of the wrap-around porch with hanging baskets, the lace curtains), hoping he would forget that he was in a snit.

It must have worked. By the time we left, he didn't know he had even been to see a doctor.

July 21, 2016

Today, while I met with eight women in my living room about an upcoming writers' conference, one of them noticed the Cadillac backing out of the driveway. That morning, I asked Troy to be sure to take the truck somewhere so Drew wouldn't be tempted to look for it while I was in the meeting. But it never occurred to me that he would go anywhere in the Cadillac since he hasn't driven it in a year or more.

I quickly assessed there was nothing I could do to catch him. It would be futile to try to chase after the car on foot or even in another car because I had no idea where he might go, and he didn't have a cell phone or wouldn't know how to answer it if he did. So I consoled myself that Drew is "an excellent driver" and said, "Let's pray." Together, we acknowledged our helplessness and asked the Lord to watch over him and bring him safely home.

Then, in a deliberate act of will, I relinquished Drew to God and turned my attention to the work at hand. The phone rang twice during the meeting, and my heart leaped into my throat both times when I glanced at the caller ID. Again and again, I forced my mind to concentrate on the details of the conference.

Then, after an hour and a half, the red car returned to the driveway, safe and sound.

As soon as the ladies dispersed, I dashed into the bedroom and said as casually as I could, "So, I see you took the Cadillac out for a little spin. Where did you wind up going?" I fully expected him to say he didn't remember.

But he did. "I went to the country club for lunch."

Later over dinner, he complained that he wasn't hungry.

"Well," I said, "that's probably because you had a late lunch. Do you remember going to the country club?"

He said he did and then told me only a few people were there and he didn't know any of them. Then he added, "It isn't any fun eating alone. I like it better when you're with me."

July 25, 2016

Drew had his six-month appointment with the cardiologist today. When the doctor asked if he remembered getting his double bypass and valve replacement operations in 2008, I could soon tell the question had more to do with his memory than his heart.

When Drew said no, the doctor pressed him. "Do you know you have a scar on your chest?"

Drew said no, and the doctor pressed again. "Do you ever take a shower and see your scar?"

Drew said, "No, we don't have a mirror in the shower." I smiled.

But the doctor wasn't done. "When you get out of the shower and look in the mirror, do you notice that you have a scar on your chest reminding you that you had heart surgery?"

"No, I don't look at my chest."

I thought that might be the end of it but . . .

"Do you remember that you had brain surgery to remove a benign tumor?"

"No."

I didn't want to say the word Alzheimer's, so I piped up with a hint: "He's taking Aricept and Namenda."

The doctor gave me a duh look. "It's not working."

We left with a good report and went to lunch at a nearby restaurant.

The hostess seated us in the middle of the room, brought us our water, and we ordered an appetizer. After she left, Drew spotted a booth at the end of the room that he liked better. "We should move over there."

"This is fine, hon. We're all settled here, and this is comfortable."

"No," he said, gathering up his silverware. "That's a better seat. Let's move."

"We can't do that. Let's ask the waitress when she comes back."

We asked her, and she replied that she would have to check with the manager.

"Why can't we just go?" Drew said. "Nobody's there."

"Let's just wait. They might not have any servers assigned to that booth."

The waitress returned and said, "I'm sorry, but that table is reserved for parties of four to six people."

I smiled and thanked her for checking while Drew scowled, held his breath in his cheeks like a pufferfish, and crossed his arms over his chest. Pouting must be a new phase. If he was going to behave like a child, I figured I would need to speak to him as a child.

Making my tone as tender as possible, I spoke softly. "I know you're disappointed, but the time to change seats is when you're first seated. Next time, let's be sure we like the place where the hostess puts us."

He continued to pout even after the food came, which he picked at. "I'm not hungry."

No amount of small talk or distractions seemed to work, so I concentrated on the salad in front of me and ate every last bite. Eventually, the waitress boxed up Drew's leftovers, and we drove home . . . where I promptly took a nap.

August 3, 2016

Last night, as Drew was sitting in his recliner in the bedroom and he said, "It's good to get away like this and have a change of scenery."

I don't know where he thought we were, but I would like to have had a glimpse of the scenery he saw at our get-away place.

I'm feeling the need for a vacation but don't know how to get one. Last week, Drew was still sleeping when I left home to go to a dental appointment, and I had this exhilarating feeling as I drove off *alone* in the car. *Ah, peace and quiet with nobody needing me.* And then I thought, *How pathetic is this—to be delighted about going to the dentist?*

In his waking hours for the past few months, Drew has been singing, "I'm gonna sit right down and write myself a letter . . . and make believe it came from you." Those are the only words he knows to the song, but he hits the notes on key. And you should see the emotion he puts into it—the loving way he points to me when he comes to the last word, "youuuu."

But I'm sick of that song. I'm tired of pretending to be enchanted by his romantic antics. I'm sick and tired of the repetition and what this disease is doing to my beloved. So I remind myself that the day may well come when I would give anything to hear him sing that stupid song to me just one more time.

August 12, 2016

This is the third week of Namenda for Drew. It's kicking in, which is a mixed bag: It's good for him because it's perked him up again, so he's sleeping less, but it's bad for me because he's shadowing me 24/7 and I'm finding it hard to concentrate on anything. A few weeks ago, when he was sleeping most of the day, I could work at the keyboard and had eased back into what felt like a normal routine with time to myself. At that point, Drew had become compliant, and I had a reprieve.

But now, we're once again at that place where Drew questions how I'm handling the finances, sits in my office and asks nonsense questions every time I try to focus on my publishing projects, and requires constant attention. I'm exhausted.

My friends Susan and Carol make it a point to meet me once a month for lunch at The Brick restaurant for encouragement, girl talk, and prayer. By the time I got done telling them how I haven't been sleeping, have mixed up a couple of appointments, and am on the verge of off and on tears because of being "tethered" to Drew, they both said, "You need to get help."

The Transitions program, a branch of Delaware Hospice, offers resources for caregivers. Before we parted, I promised to look into it. I found their number online, but it took a couple of days for me to be able to find "alone time" to make the call. It turns out that I already knew Al Morris, so I felt right at home when we spoke on the phone.

We set up an appointment for the 18th at the CHEER Center so he could fill me in on what resources they offer. Because Drew doesn't think there's anything wrong with him, he wouldn't understand volunteers coming to the house to be with him. So I don't know how this will work out, but at least I'm connecting with "hope."

In the meantime, I have a strong network of praying friends who call and frequently e-mail to let me know they are interceding for me. I like it best when they pray with me over the phone, such as tonight when Barry Jones and Elizabeth Boerner felt led to call.

The way I see it,
if you want the rainbow,
you gotta put up with the rain.

— Dolly Parton

CHAPTER SIXTEEN

Goodbye Mild Stage, Hello Moderate

August 18, 2016

I met with Al to talk about the Transitions program this morning, and what a treasure trove of information he had to offer. One of the first things he said is that there is no charge. He guided me through a thorough review of the Delaware Hospice care, and I signed a paper to get Drew enrolled for the full range of services, beginning with the Transitions program, which is designed for caregivers. (See Appendix for more information on Delaware Hospice.)

Al informed me that since hospice care has become such a competitive field, several others in Sussex County also provide similar services, which I may or may not look into. I asked if this type of care is provided nationwide, and he replied that each state offers hospice care but under different names and guidelines.

He sent me home with a full packet of resources—everything from matching us up with volunteers who would help with grocery shopping to transportation and options for respite care. The packet included a copy of James L. Miller's two-sided book. One side was entitled, *When You're the Caregiver: 12 Things To Do If Someone You Care For Is Ill or Incapacitated*; and the flip side (intentionally printed upside down) is called *When You're Ill or Incapacitated: 12 Things To Remember in Times of Sickness, Injury, or Disability.* (See Appendix for other books I've found helpful.)

I got a tour of the adult day care facility at the CHEER Center, which has activities for all levels of aptitude as well as a porch for fresh-air days. Drew wouldn't be receptive to going at this point because he's a private person. In fact, his definition of success is "being master of your own time" and not having to be anywhere by a certain time. But as things change, I can see us giving it a try a little later on. After all, ever since I've known him, he has disliked cucumbers, but now he eats them. Why? Because he forgot he doesn't like them. So maybe adult day care will be something we can take advantage of in due time.

Al and I talked about the importance of exercise—Drew's and mine—and how even a short walk (ten minutes one way and ten minutes back), would do us good. I'm looking forward to cooler weather so Drew and I can do that.

An interesting thing happened during my conversation with Al, who shared about his own experience with burnout as a caretaker and the consequences for his health. When I first sat down with him, my whole body felt like a clock that had been wound too tightly to function. By the time I left, my hands swung looser by my side, and I could feel my face glowing. Nothing had changed except for the comfort I received from someone who not only knew what I'm facing but also provided tangible options for taking better care of myself.

Tonight at dusk, Drew took Buttercup out and then poked his head inside the house and said, "You need to come out here." I half grunted because I had just settled into my recliner and wanted to rest. But that's exactly what he had in mind. He wanted me to rest with him in our rocking chairs in the calm of the evening with the gentle breeze caressing our cheeks and the birds chirping.

The temperature was perfect, and it didn't take long for me to recognize the golden opportunity before me. I turned on the little fountain to add the sound of babbling water, but something was still missing: music.

I dashed inside and got my Kindle and a portable speaker. It only took a second to press the Pandora radio app, locate our favorite "Letterman" station, and adjust the volume. Soft, nostalgic chords and harmonious voices filled the air as the hues in the sky changed to streaks of pink and orange, adding a healthy glow to Drew's contented face. Buttercup and Midnight, our indoor/outdoor black cat, paced around and finally settled by our feet.

Five or ten minutes passed and Drew entertained himself by looking for jet streams, pointing out airplanes, and guessing at their destinations. I picked up my Kindle and immersed myself in the pages of a book. Because the pages are backlit, I didn't realize that it had gotten dark until Drew said, "Look at that moon." It was full and *huge*.

I half expected him to ask me to run and get the camera, but he didn't. I closed my Kindle, and we sat there admiring the shining globe and talking softly about how blessed we are. Gratitude flowed from both of us for the privacy of our backyard; the good, kind neighbors we have; our gentle-natured pets; the freedoms we have in America; and the joy of having each other.

All in all, we spent about an hour and a half on the deck, which was more satisfying to me than a week's vacation.

August 31, 2016

Another decline has crept up on us—more abilities going by the wayside.

Drew needed to sign his formal name, Andrew C. Abbott, so I had him practice. At first, he tackled it casually, concentrating on hooking the capital A with the "n" for Andrew. But his brow quickly became furrowed, and after six or seven tries, a panicky look came over him.

"I can sign for you," I said, and the relief that washed over him was overpowering. It made me wish I had offered sooner, but now I know for sure that he can no longer sign anything official.

He's having more trouble than usual remembering normal household things. He asked where we keep the ". . . you know, the thing that we . . ." and went through some hand gyrations, pointing in the direction of the kitchen and trying to gesture wiping a counter. I figured out he was asking about paper towels and directed him to the closet where we keep paper products. You can imagine the wave of sadness that swept over me ten minutes later when I found the empty paper towel tube still in its holder and a roll of toilet tissue sitting on the countertop. He wants so badly to help around the house like he always did, but his memory keeps short-circuiting and sabotaging him.

He went into the bathroom to shave and then came to get me and asked, "Where is my shaving stuff?" (which was sitting conspicuously on the vanity by the sink).

I picked up the razor, put it in his right hand, and smiled. "Here you go. This is your razor, and"—holding up the can—"this is your shaving cream."

"It was there all the time?" he wanted to know.

"Yep, right there, hiding in plain sight."

From that point on, he was fine and able to shave.

September 7, 2016

Namenda may be making him more alert, but it sure isn't helping with his memory. For the past four or five nights, while lying in our bed and about to go to sleep, he's peppered me with questions that make it clear he doesn't recognize his own home: "Who owns this place?" "I guess we leave tomorrow, right?" "When this thing docks (or parks), where will we be?"

I tell him he's at home, right where he belongs, but the questions continue. "You say we're in Georgetown, but where is this place located?" "How'd we get here?" "Who's taking care of the dogs?"

"We are," I say. "But we only have one dog and one cat. Buttercup is right behind the chair in her bed, and Midnight is outside."

I can still hear him fretting and jibber-jabbering as I doze off around midnight or 1:00 a.m. One night it was 2:00, and he was still going strong trying to figure it out. Since he's never been much of a traveler, I find it strange that he's stuck in an "away from home" mindset. But then, his home where things are "normal" doesn't look normal to him through the fog of Alzheimer's. So far, the best thing I've come up with to say is, "All you need to know is you're in a safe place with someone who loves you, and everything's fine." That makes him chuckle, and soon the questions end for the night.

September 9, 2016

So many things to think about—all the time. Today is one of those days when I'd like to stop the world and get off, but there's too much to be done.

We found a buyer for the Bedford Motors building, and settlement is scheduled for October 24th, but you know what the paperwork trail is like on this sort of thing.

I'm still trying to sort out the new revocable trust situation with the elder law attorney, so I'm surrounded by piles of legalese . . . while trying to keep the bills current. In fact, I just found a bill from Lowe's buried under some papers on Drew's desk that was due August 20th. I hope that doesn't affect our credit score.

I tried to listen for the mail truck yesterday, but he beat me to it and came to me with a frown on his face. "What's this?" He had opened the attorney's bill for the deed preparation they're doing for me.

I had to do a quick two-step around that one. "Let's go to dinner," I said, "and I'll tell you all about it." It worked. By the time we got into the car, he had forgotten all about it.

Publishing is going wild around here, too. I'm working with four new authors and am trying to give each one of them the attention they deserve. This is a happy problem, and fortunately, all my clients are very understanding.

I had intended to go to a funeral yesterday (a praying friend who no longer struggles with cancer) and another today (the husband of a praying friend who died suddenly from a heart attack). Both services are being held at the same church an hour away, but I don't want to be away from Drew for three hours—so here I am, feeling guilty. But I won't dwell on it because, as I am often reminded, I need to take care of myself, and it gives me peace to be at home tending to the things that could easily get out of balance.

September 12, 2016

I noticed a change over the weekend regarding Drew's ability to be responsive, but it didn't fully register until today. When our grandson, Kade, hugged him on Saturday, he sat in the chair and received the hug but didn't make any effort to hug him back. Yesterday Dana stopped in for a visit. Drew didn't stand up as he usually does when she was ready to leave, so she leaned down and hugged him. Although he smiled and said, "See you, hon," he didn't hug her in return. This is just another sign that he is counting on others to do everything for him with little to no effort on his part.

Today I met with my friend and publishing client, Pam Halter, in Smyrna, which is about halfway for both of us, an hour and a half or so. Drew stayed home alone with Buttercup. (I wrote a note on a dry erase board on the bar with my phone number, and Troy checked in on him.) When I got home, I found the dog food bowl full of kibble saturated with a sickly-looking something-or-other. It seems he poured a can of chocolate Boost on it to make it more appetizing. Good thing Buttercup didn't like it because chocolate is bad for dogs. It's sad when a man can't even feed his dog.

Pam brought me bags of fresh Jersey produce—tomatoes, corn, cantaloupes, and nectarines. I also picked up some shrimp salad from a seafood place on the way home, so tonight I cooked.

I counted the times Drew said, "Excellent meal." Twenty-five. Now, that kind of repetition I can take. It might even motivate me to cook more often.

September 20, 2016

Twice now, about two weeks apart, Drew opened his mouth to say something, and gibberish came out. Both times, his eyes expressed alarm, as if to say, "What just happened?" Fortunately, his normal speech resumed immediately afterward on those occasions.

The first time this happened was in a restaurant while the waitress was taking our order. It reminded me of last spring when Drew said, "I just came in from China, and I don't speak English." But this time, his speech was more like, "Keeynomsobbybobbobchumsey." The waitress's head jerked back, and she looked as startled as Drew did.

"You just never know what's going to pop out of him," I said. "He's just trying to be funny."

Then I turned to Drew. "I don't think they have that on the menu today." And we all got a good belly laugh out of it.

This isn't really funny because I think it's a sign that he's slipping deeper into the moderate phase. I've noticed that when a shift is about to occur in his decline, a symptom will happen once and I'll ignore it. When it happens a second time, I pay attention. After that, I know to expect the same symptom to occur more frequently until it eventually becomes commonplace.

The leader of our support group says there's a psychiatric term for this sort of babbling gobbledygook: "word salad." It's defined as "a confused or unintelligible mixture of seemingly random words and phrases."

Word salad. This, coming from the man whose words have comforted and consoled me over these many years. Gibberish from the man who told me on our first date, "You look like a woman who needs to be appreciated," and has been doing just that ever since.

So now, it's my turn to appreciate him, more than ever before, as we navigate our way through unknown territory known as the moderate phase.

Every evening I turn my worries over to God.
He's going to be up all night anyway.

—Mary C. Crowley

CHAPTER SEVENTEEN
Who Is He, Really?

Moderate phase. "Moderate." Now, there is a word less apt to describe Drew if I've ever heard one—even if it is clinical.

Drew was named Andrew Clive. He never could figure out why his mother would give him a middle name like that. He asked her one night as we were gathered around her dining room table with his brothers and the rest of the family while eating roast beef, mixed vegetables, and snow-whipped potatoes.

"Mom, why would you hang a name like Clive on an unsuspecting infant? Was I named after somebody, or does it have some special meaning?"

She placed her finger on the side of her chin and gazed at the ceiling while we waited in anticipation. Tilting her head, she spoke at last. "I can't remember."

"You give somebody a name like that and then can't remember why?" We all cracked up.

But his first name was most appropriate. Drew, short for Andrew, in many ways, developed into his biblical namesake. Andrew, Simon Peter's brother, was the humble one who submitted himself to Jesus. Andrew's hallmark was his unwavering faith. Yes, Drew has the right name. I think of my Drew as humble and faithful to God, to me—and to so many people.

Who is Drew Abbott, really? An eighty-year-old man who is declining with Alzheimer's and approaching number five out of eight stages? Yes. But he is so much more.

He is the little boy who was happy to be quarantined with scarlet fever because it meant that he and his big brother, Howard, could stay home and play with toy soldiers all day long.

He is the first-grade student about whom his teacher wrote, "Keeps his hands to himself."

He is the kid who had a dog named Trixie and a pony named Dolly and then grew up to become the man who loves dogs, cats, squirrels, and bunnies—but hates snakes.

He is the son who never complained when his mother made him take piano lessons.

He is the son who adored his father and followed in his footsteps as a car dealer and owner of rental properties.

He is the high school student whose strong legs set a state record for the 50-yard dash.

He is Tim and Dean's older brother who could easily distance himself when his two siblings tormented each other.

He is the youngster who attended Georgetown Presbyterian Church before his feet could touch the floor, and he claimed the same pew for the rest of his life.

He is the teenager who just got his license and was stopped by a cop when he was following his softball buddies out of state.

"The light was yellow," Drew told the policeman.

The officer pulled himself up to full height, which made him look like a giant. "When a Philadelphia cop says it's red, it's red."

Drew nodded. "Yes, sir. May I say something?"

The officer nodded. "Go ahead."

Drew pointed. "You see those cars just pulling out of sight over that hill?"

"Yeah. What about it?"

"Well, I'm following them, and if I don't catch up soon, I'll *never* find my way home."

The cop smiled ever so slightly. "Go ahead. But son, be careful."

He is the football running back who married his high school sweetheart, but she left him later for another man.

He is the president of the Georgetown High School class of 1954 and the one his classmates still look up to.

He is the "greatest dad in the world" according to Dana and Troy, as well as the single parent who kept the household secure until I came along to help out.

He is Kim's stepdad, who raised her from the time she was three-and-a-half years old and has so much in common with her that they could be blood-related.

He is the councilman who served for twenty-two years in the 3rd Ward in Georgetown and rode in Return Day parades after every election.

He is the golfer who was a charter member of the Sussex Pines Country Club, where he enjoyed pitchers of beer and lots of laughs with Harold McCabe, Jimmy Walls, and Linford Faucett.

He is the soldier in the Delaware National Guard whose sergeant once left him in charge of his pet monkey. Drew fed him slices of an apple through the cage until the monkey grabbed the knife and put it sideways into his mouth. Oh, my God, he's gonna kill himself! he thought, but he tricked the monkey into spitting it out.

He is the car salesman who treated people right and had loyal customers who, to this day, remember those Pontiac/GMC Truck days with fondness.

He is the one who took over Bedford Motors at thirty-two years of age after his dad's unexpected death and had to fight a panic attack on his way to sign the papers with General Motors.

He is the granddad who doted on Natalie and raised Trevor like a son, attending more Little League games than we could keep track of, including the state championship that went all the way to Bristol, Connecticut.

He is the granddad who, while riding with Kim, Wyatt, Kade, Saige, and me enjoyed a dining car experience of *The Polar Express*. On the way home, he was relieved to learn that the passenger seat of their vehicle was heated because he thought his "butt had a fever."

He is the Mr. Fix-it who never saw a gadget that he couldn't figure out or save—even if it couldn't be fixed.

He is the detail-oriented certified residential appraiser who preferred estate planning appraisals over drive-by ones because of his compassion for grieving families.

He is a gentleman, filled with problem-solving solutions, who was depended on by many—especially me.

CHAPTER EIGHTEEN

Refined as Gold

It seems like almost every family I know is dealing with some intensely stressful situation. For some, it's a matter of life and death; for others, it's mental or emotional turmoil or financial desperation. It's brought me to this conclusion: these trials we're going through are the "refining fires" that the Lord has ordained for each of us.

My new perspective is to submit myself to these fires, however long they last and however intense they get, trusting in Christ to get me through them so that I will come out on the other side refined as gold. Zechariah 13:9 (KJV) says,

> And I will bring the third part through the fire, and will refine
> them as silver is refined, and will try them as gold is tried:
> they shall call on my name, and I will hear them: I will say,
> It is my people: and they shall say, The Lord is my God.

Christ is coming back for His bride (the body of believers), and I've always wondered how He would transform this raggedy bunch of misfits that is "the church" into a bride that is spotless and pure.

> Christ loved the church and gave himself up for her to make her holy . . . to present her to himself as a radiant church, without stain or wrinkle or any other blemish, but holy and blameless (Ephesians 5:25b-27 NIV).

Everything in us cries out for relief, an escape hatch, but that's not the answer. If Christ thinks my character needs to be refined, then I don't want to try to wiggle out of it before the work He's doing in me is finished. Over the years, I have often prayed that the Lord would make and mold me into His image. If I'm sincere about this and Alzheimer's is the chisel He has chosen to use, dare I whine and question the Master?

Another way to look at the same concept is by considering how the silversmith works. He melts the silver, and the impurities rise to the surface so he can skim them off. When he can clearly see his reflection in the silver pool, he knows it's pure. The Lord also wants us to reflect His image. When we harbor frustration, bitterness, or resentment, these "impurities" hinder the transformation God is working within us. Caregiving and other trying situations have a way of exposing these traits in us.

The longer we practice "righteous indignation" or however else we justify our negative thoughts and behavior, the longer we will stay in the melting pot. This is our chance to take control of something. We can choose to forgive instead of letting our offenses fester and produce more impurities. Only then will the Father be able to see His reflection when He gazes upon us.

And let's not forget the potter and the clay. Everybody knows that the potter puts the ceramic piece into the kiln, where it is fired to a temperature high enough to solidify the clay. Did you know that when it cools, the potter pings the lip to see if it sings? If it doesn't, that tells him it's not ready, and back into the fire it goes.

Applying this analogy to us, what we're going through in taking care of a loved one with Alzheimer's isn't punishment or torture but an opportunity to grow in maturity, patience, and compassion. Any complaints we have, no matter how justified, only hold us back from realizing the joy that comes from selfless service to others and an appreciation of their value as human beings fashioned in the image of God.

Do we love only the lovable? Someone once said, "The person who is the most unlovable is the one who needs love the most." I think this is a test of our capacity to love as God loves and to learn to praise Him in the midst of it for helping us through our days.

I'm already becoming a stronger, kinder, better-balanced person because of this experience, yet I still have a lot to go through in my Alzheimer's journey with Drew. However, I'm quicker to recognize when I need an attitude adjustment, and often it boils down to confessing, "Lord, make me willing," or "Lord, help me do this because I can't do it on my own." In laying down all control and trusting God to do for me what I can't do on my own, there is freedom.

Knowing there is a purpose to this and holding on to the hope of a good outcome makes this trial easier to bear. In fact, keeping a heavenly viewpoint has led me to a "sweet spot" of true, unwavering peace. Nothing has changed on the outside—just my attitude on the inside. The key is maintaining this perspective and staying alert to avoid traps that would derail me . . . like having to answer the same question for the twenty-fourth time.

When the kids were young and our household was bustling with other worries and a different kind of stress, Drew used to ask me this question: "Can you handle this moment?" I would stop whatever I was doing and take inventory of THIS moment. Can I stand here in the front yard and appreciate this gentle breeze and birds chirping?

POOF! That moment is gone.

Can I handle this moment? Yes. Whatever "this" moment is, the Lord promises strength not only to endure but to overcome. At this moment, I can seek out comfort from others. I can talk over this "unsolvable puzzle" with someone who can offer wisdom. I can search the Scriptures for God's perspective on this very moment. The Lord reminds me of how often He has gotten me through difficult times before, and He will be faithful tomorrow, showing me how to do "the next thing" no matter how difficult it may be.

So ask yourself, "Can I handle this moment?" If you're tempted to answer no, invite the Lord to handle "this moment" for you.

The goal is peace—peace in this moment. And with the Holy Spirit's help, you can find it.

Be joyful in hope, patient in affliction, faithful in prayer.
—Romans 12:12 (NIV)

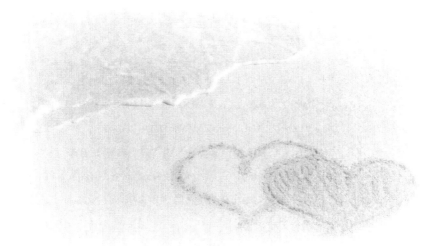

Epilogue

My journey with Drew continues as we slip deeper into the moderate phase and then, if Alzheimer's follows its natural progression, into the severe phase. From my growing library of resources, I have an idea of what lies ahead—coping with his severe mood changes; adjusting to the probability of him not recognizing me and eventually being unable to speak; learning how to care for him when he grows incontinent; scheduling an array of respite care workers, nurses, and volunteers; and making end-of-life decisions.

I'll keep writing about our journey, but a lot of people have encouraged me to share this much now because "people need to know." Assured that Drew wouldn't recognize himself if he happened to see the cover, I have taken the plunge in releasing these pages to the public. I hope you have found them informative, enlightening, inspirational, or entertaining if you are trying to find your way through this maze of what is sometimes called the "caregiver's disease."

In the meantime, I will concentrate on the moments in front of me, like Drew's playfulness last night while we were eating our turkey sandwiches on toasted rye at Pizza Palace. He belched loud enough for everyone to hear, not once but three times in quick succession, and then gave me an ornery grin.

Remembering my mother's admonition when my brothers were little, "Don't encourage him," I pretended not to notice.

When I told him he had a crumb on his lip, he wiped his face with a napkin everywhere but where he knew the crumb was located.

Again, I forced myself to keep a straight face and ignored the silliness.

Then, he put a French fry in his mouth and left most of it hanging out so it dangled like a cigar, bobbing up and down as he chewed.

This time, using my best deadpan look (think Alice and Ralph on Jackie Gleason's "The Honeymooners"), I said in a monotone voice, "You're really fun to be around."

He laughed and shoved the rebellious French fry into his mouth. As he chewed, a crimson color crept up his neck and into his cheeks.

"You're blushing," I said and laughed with him.

The color deepened, proving that he still knows what it feels like to get caught doing something he's not supposed to do, that his sense of humor is still intact, and he and I are still fully engaged in life.

I've never loved him more.

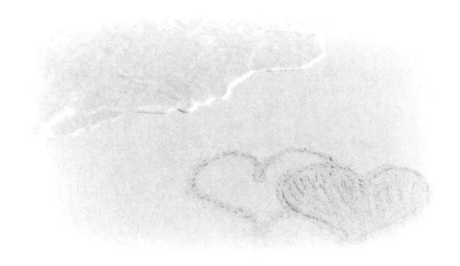

Meet the Author

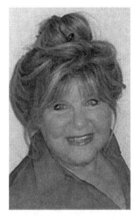

Candy Abbott is a wife, grandmom, author, publisher, and inspirational speaker. Most of all, she considers herself a "fruitbearer" because it is her life's goal to exhibit the fruit of the Spirit as described in Galatians 5:22-23 (love, joy, peace, patience, kindness, goodness, faithfulness, gentleness, and self-control). Candy's award-winning independent publishing company, Fruitbearer Publishing LLC, was established in 1999. She founded Delmarva Christian Writers' Fellowship (www.delmarvawriters.com) and Mothers With a Mission (www.motherswithamission.org). Candy lives in Georgetown, Delaware, with her husband, Drew, their Cocker Spaniel, Buttercup, and their black cat, Midnight. They have three children, four grandchildren, and became great-grandparents in 2017, with another on the way. For more information, visit www.fruitbearer.com.

Never be afraid to trust
an unknown future
to a known God.

—Corrie ten Boom

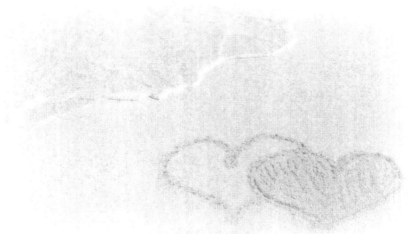

Resources I've Found Helpful

The 36-Hour Day, 5th edition: A Family Guide to Caring for People Who Have Alzheimer Disease, Related Dementias, and Memory Loss by Peter V. Rabins and Nancy L Mace.

Caregiving Our Loved Ones: Stories and Strategies That Will Change Your Life by Nanette J. Davis, Ph.D.

Understand Alzheimer's: A First-Time Caregiver's Plan to Understand and Prepare for Alzheimer's & Dementia by Kevin Pierce, Calistoga Press.

Chicken Soup for the Caregiver's Soul: Stories to Inspire Caregivers in the Home, the Community and the World by Jack Canfield (author), Mark Victor Hansen (author), LeAnn Thieman L.P.N. (author).

Songs You Know By Heart: A Simple Guide for Using Music in Dementia Care by Mary Sue Wilkinson with contributions by Teepa Snow and the companion CD from www.singinghearttoheart.com.

Learning to Speak Alzheimer's: A Groundbreaking Approach for Everyone Dealing with the Disease by Joanne Koenig Coste with the foreword by Robert N. Butler, M.D.

My Turn to Care: Encouragement for Caregivers of Aging Parents by Marlene Bagnull.

When You're the Caregiver: 12 Things To Do If Someone You Care For Is Ill or Incapacitated by James L. Miller. The flip side (intentionally printed upside down) is, *When You're Ill or Incapacitated: 12 Things To Remember in Times of Sickness, Injury, or Disability.*

The Loss of Self: A Family Resource for the Care of Alzheimer's Disease and Related Disorders by Donna Cohen, Ph.D. and Carl Eisdorfer, Ph.D., M.D.

A Promise Kept: The Story of an Unforgettable Love by Robertson McQuilkin.

Free DVD, *The Senior Gems,* from Senior Helpers. Request a free, informative DVD, "Your Guide to Supporting Family Members with Dementia," featuring Teepa Snow. http://www.seniorhelpers.com/services/senior-gems.

Visit www.alzstore.com for innovative toys, safety products, and a wealth of information.

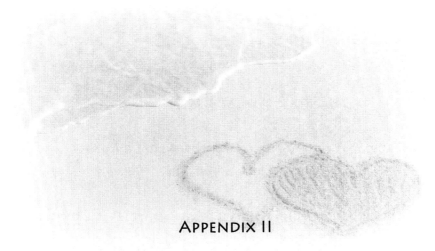

ONE OF MANY TIPS FROM ALZ.ORG

Rummaging, Hiding, and Hoarding Behaviors

Persons with dementia experience memory loss, mental confusion, disorientation, impaired judgment and behavioral changes. One of these changes may include "hoarding." While hoarding is often harmless, it can become a health and safety issue for the person with dementia.

Some people are natural "collectors" who have accumulated things that are important to them over the years. They may have difficulty getting rid of items because of the personal meaning they hold. Hoarding for a person with dementia may be more likely to happen in the early and middle stages of dementia and often stems from trying to have some control in their lives. People with dementia may be driven to search or rummage for something that they believe is missing.

Possible Causes
Psychological or Medical Causes

- Physical changes in the brain cause memory loss, impaired judgment, and confusion

- Inability to remember taking items, unable to remember where the items were placed or hidden

- Loss of control over behaviors

- Rummaging, hiding, and hoarding are all things an individual does to gain a sense of security. For example, individuals may hoard items out of fear that they may "need" the items someday. Individuals may begin to hide items when they are not able to recognize the people around them any longer. Individuals may rummage through items because seeing and touching the items reminds them that they are there and gives them comfort.

- Environmental causes

- Fear of being robbed or losing items; hiding or hoarding items in an attempt to make them safe

- Inability to distinguish between items that should be kept or thrown away

- Lack of stimulation, boredom, or difficulty initiating new activities.

Coping Strategies
Addressing Clutter and Hoarding

In most cases removing all clutter can cause severe emotional upset, and it is usually not beneficial to remove everything that a person hoards. This is because the items that the person collects give them a sense of security and safety. Also, individuals may have emotional attachments to items that appear to others to be worthless or useless.

When removing clutter:

- Only remove what is needed to eliminate safety and health hazards. Leave behind as much safe clutter as you can. Organize it in large bins or baskets away from walking pathways, stairs, stoves, and heaters.

- Give the individual a good reason to part with their items. They may be more willing to let go of something if they are told that the item will be given to a charity, church, family member, etc.

- Negotiate. Trade a year's worth of newspapers for a month's worth. Trade rotten or expired food for fresh food.

- Be creative. Take pictures of items that are given away, and allow the person to keep the pictures. Allow the person to take the time to say goodbye to items that you may perceive as worthless.

- Remove discarded items immediately because the person may rummage through the garbage and bring items back into their home.

- If the individual agrees to help de-clutter, give them one box of items to sort through at a time. Start slowly and take breaks frequently.

- Be prepared for the person's reaction and have support for the person and yourself. You may want to involve family, friends, clergy, or a social worker. Have activities planned and ready to divert the person's attention from the removal of their items.

- Reduce the amount of clutter coming into the home by reducing spending money and monitoring purchases. Consider blocking home shopping channels. Stop junk mail and catalog mailings by visiting www.dmachoice.org, www.catalogchoice.org, and www.optoutprescreen.com. Consider getting bills sent to another address, if needed.

- What you view as cluttered and disorganized may help the individual function and cope. Some individuals keep belongings out in the open or in unusual places because they may forget where they are if they cannot see them. If the clutter is not posing a safety or health hazard, then leave it as is.

Make Rummaging Productive

- Restricting access to all drawers and cabinets can be distressing for a person who enjoys rummaging. Many individuals will rummage or constantly reorganize items because they feel a need to be productive.

- Provide the individual with an opportunity to rummage and make rummaging a stimulating activity. This can be done by providing easy access to some closets, drawers, or portable boxes that contain safe items that the individual can rummage in. They can contain random items or be themed: sewing drawer, sports closet, jewelry box, etc.

- If the individual enjoys sorting and organizing items, do this activity. Ask the person to help you fold and sort items like socks, napkins, and scarves. This may help the person fulfill their desire to be productive.

If God sends us on stony paths,
He will provide us with strong shoes.

—Alexander MacLaren

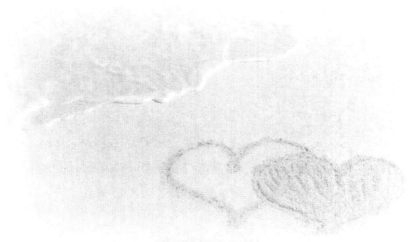

DELAWARE HOSPICE

(Check for similar programs in your state or county.)

The Four Stages of Care

Transitions. The Transitions program provides guidance and resources to families coping with a serious illness. It's for families that may not be ready for hospice yet.

- Offers non-medical support for people coping with a serious illness such as heart disease, stroke, Alzheimer's, cancer, Parkinson's, liver and lung disease, or kidney failure
- Regular contact overseen by a Transitions Coordinator
- Identification of appropriate community resources
- Assistance with lifestyle changes
- Trained volunteers who can provide companionship, assistance, and/or transportation
- Can be customized depending on your needs, at no charge

Delaware Palliative.

Palliative care helps families cope with the physical and psychosocial burdens of a serious illness through home visits by a physician, nurse practitioner, and a social worker. Palliative focuses on the human side.

- Helps seriously ill patients who are receiving active curative treatment for illnesses such as cancer, congestive heart failure, Parkinson's, Alzheimer's, and kidney failure

- Offers symptom management support to seriously ill people who are not terminally ill

- Appropriate from the time an illness has been diagnosed, throughout treatment, and the final stages of the disease

- Provides comfort, clarity, choice, and connections

- Covered by Medicare Part B, Medicaid, and most private insurance plans, and copays, co-insurance, and deductibles may apply

Delaware Hospice.

The Hospice program focuses on meeting the physical, emotional, and spiritual needs of patients and families with life-limiting illnesses through the care of a multi-disciplinary team.

- Supports and educates patients and their caregivers as they navigate end-of-life care

- Travels to the patient at their residence, nursing homes, assisted living facilities, or even hospitals

- Covered by Medicare Part A, Medicaid, and most private insurance plans

The Delaware Hospice Center.
Though hospice provides services wherever you may call home, there are times when your loved one may need a higher level of care than they can get at home. The Delaware Hospice Center is an alternative to going to the hospital, keeping patients comfortable and safe when symptoms or pain arise.

- Offers a higher level of specialized 24-hour care to hospice patients who require symptom management

- Respite care also an option for patients and their caregivers

- Available to those who qualify for Delaware Hospice

- Covered by Medicare Part A, Medicaid, and most private insurance plans

They may forget what you said,
but they will never forget
how you made them feel.

— Carl W. Buechner

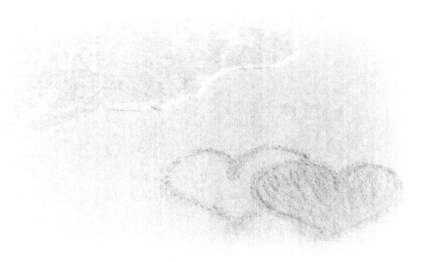

Order Info

I've Never Loved Him More
is available from
Amazon or wherever books are sold.

For autographed copies,
visit www.fruitbearer.com
or contact Candy
at info@fruitbearer.com
302.856.6649

Fruitbearer Publishing LLC
P.O. Box 777, Georgetown, DE 19947

Candy's Other Books

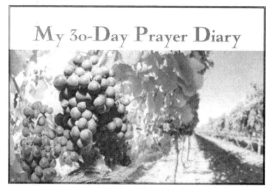

MY 30-DAY PRAYER DIARY

This handy diary is was created as a companion to *Fruitbearer: What Can I Do for You, Lord?* by Candy Abbott. It is patterned after the prayer diary by Catherine Marshall and Leonard LeSourd that Candy used in her journey to become better acquainted with the Holy Spirit. Come near to God, and He will come near to you (James 4:8) is a promise from His holy Word. By committing yourself to thirty days of prayer, you are intentionally drawing near to God, and you can do so in confidence, knowing that He is drawing near. Many of the topics addressed in this diary will be familiar, probably all of them, but each time these areas confront our spirit, we may be in a different frame of mind or circumstance. The blank portion, "My Prayer Requests" and "God's Answers" can be used to record your own personal spiritual journey or prayer concerns for others. If the Holy Spirit speaks to your heart, capture His words and date the entry so you can reflect on them later. The Word is alive in those of us who believe. Give the Holy Spirit freedom to search areas you may have resisted before.

SPIRIT FRUIT: A CANDID CALENDAR FOR FRUITFUL LIVING

This perpetual calendar will tickle your funny bone, make you think, and strengthen your spirit. A light and unexpected approach to biblical and everyday truths, *Spirit Fruit* will become your daily friend and be a good conversation piece for the whole family . . . year after year.

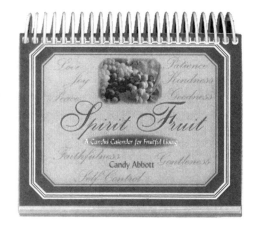

Candy's Other Books

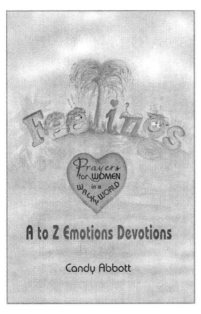

FEELINGS: PRAYERS FOR WOMEN IN A WACKY WORLD

A TO Z EMOTIONS DEVOTIONS

Are your emotions soaring heavenward one minute and splashing for survival the next? This devotional will keep you anchored in Scripture so you can hear God's voice and heed His call, whether you're sinking or swimming. Each "feelings" page begins with "Lord, I feel _____," followed by a real-life situation, a relevant Scripture, and the Lord's perspective. Try it yourself. Half of the pages are lined for you to journal your own feelings.

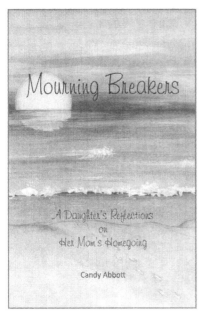

MOURNING BREAKERS: A DAUGHTER'S REFLECTIONS ON HER MOM'S HOMEGOING

Tears may flow in the night, but joy comes in the morning (Psalm 30:5).

If you are grieving the loss of a loved one or helping someone through their final days on earth, this brief personal experience devotional is a proven resource for caretakers who are seeking an anchor. Find your joy in the mourning.

Candy's Other Books

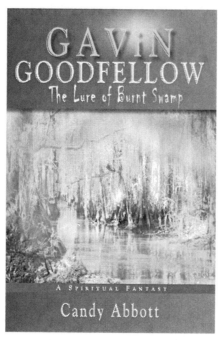

GAVIN GOODFELLOW: THE LURE OF BURNT SWAMP

What do twelve-year-old dyslexic Gavin Goodfellow, prophetically-inclined Uncle Warney, mother-daughter witches from London, and a tattooed New Age guru have in common? Burnt Swamp—where flames from a mysterious underground fire have been smoldering for ten years. The battle is on for dominion of the swamp and possession of an ancient diary that holds clues to release or destroy the evil that dwells beneath the surface. Will Gavin respond to the Holy Spirit and embrace his God-given calling? Or will Bea Daark and her mum unleash forces that lure Gavin and the sleepy town of Ashboro deep into bondage?

Book One of the Burnt Swamp Trilogy

"Just when I thought the best fantasy-mystery-adventure books had already been written, I found *Gavin Goodfellow*. NOW you have the best! Not only is the story deliciously strange and can't-put-it-down intriguing, but Gavin and the challenges he bumps into are as real as you are. And at the center of it all, there's God—like you've never experienced God before. So follow Gavin and his cousins, Molly and Eric, into Burnt Swamp and be prepared for the journey of your life!"

—Nancy Rue, award-winning author
of youth and adult fiction

Candy's First Book

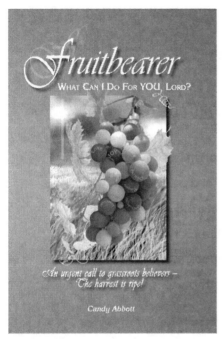

FRUITBEARER: WHAT CAN I DO FOR YOU, LORD?

If you've ever cried out, "Help me, Jesus!", or "Use me, Lord!" then you are in a good position to become a fruitbearer. If you've ever responded to God's call when it made no sense, then you may already be a fruitbearer. If you hunger for a closer relationship with God, then you will be inspired by Candy Abbott's journey from a casual believer to a bonafide, undisputed fruitbearer.

With back-to-back natural disasters, financial stress, global chaos, and personal trials at every turn, it is more important than ever to trust Christ to empower you for service. Consider this a guidebook to fruitful living in a sour grape society. Invite the Holy Spirit to speak to you between the lines of these pages, and you will discover a new depth and fresh appreciation for Christ's work in your life. Rather than ask, "What can God do for me?" let the Holy Spirit prompt you to ask, "What can I do for YOU, Lord?"

Fruitbearer is the book for you:

- if you long for the excitement the early Christians experienced and want to produce lasting fruit for the Kingdom of God;
- if you long for the power to live your faith joyfully and make God your top priority;
- if you long to recognize the voice of the Holy Spirit and sense a "call" on your life but feel inadequate;
- if you long to have Christ's peace, even in the midst of turmoil, so you can impart peace to others.

249

With Gratitude

This book has the fingerprints and heart-prints
of many who prayed. helped me along the way,
and are helping me still.
Consider this a blanket thank you
for the love, support, and skills
generously shared and eternally appreciated.

Candy

CPSIA information can be obtained
at www.ICGtesting.com
Printed in the USA
LVOW10s1655151117

556257LV00021B/1452/P